THE BEST CHAFFLES RECIPES 2021

EASY TASTY LOW CARB AND GLUTEN-FREE KETOGENIC WAFFLES TO BOOST FAT BURNING, LOSE WEIGHT AND IMPROVE YOUR HEALTH BY EATING DELICIOUS FOOD

Tables of contents

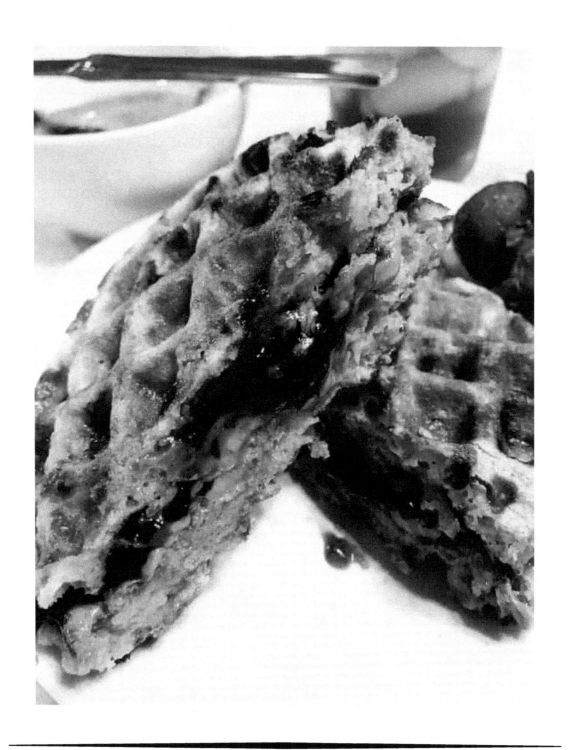

INTRODUCTION

The ketogenic diet is a high-fat, low-carb diet that keeps on account of how effectively it can assist you with arriving at your health and wellness objectives. In any case, numerous individuals, despite everything, need the keto diet.

The ketogenic diet — most usually alluded to just as "keto" — is a high-fat, low-carbohydrate diet that places your body in a fat-consuming state known as ketosis. In ketosis, your body utilizes muscle versus fat, as opposed to carbs, as its principle wellspring of vitality.

To get into a condition of ketosis, chopping down your carb admission is imperative. Numerous individuals think about the keto diet as an overly high-fat diet, yet devouring monstrous measures of fat isn't so significant as slicing carbs with regards to changing your digestion to run on fat.

At the centre of the great keto diet is seriously limiting admission of all or most foods with sugar and starch (carbohydrates). These foods are separated into sugar (insulin and glucose) in our blood once we eat them, and if these levels become excessively high, additional calories are significantly more effortlessly stored as muscle to fat ratio and result in undesirable weight gain. Nonetheless, when glucose levels are sliced off because of low-carb consumption, the body begins to consume fat instead and produces some ketones that can be estimated in the blood (utilizing pee strips, for instance).

Keto diets, like most of the low carb diets, work through the end of glucose. Since a lot of people live on a high carb diet, our bodies regularly run on glucose (or sugar) for vitality. We can't cause glucose and just to have around 24 hours' worth stored in our muscle tissue and liver. When glucose is never again accessible from food sources, we start to consume stored fat rather, or fat from our food.

Subsequently, when you're following a ketogenic diet plan for tenderfoots, your body is consuming fat for vitality instead of carbohydrates, so in the process, the vast majority lose weight and overabundance muscle to fat ratio quickly, in any event, when expending loads of fat and satisfactory calories through their everyday food consumption. Other advantage of the keto diet is that there's no compelling reason to tally calories, feel hungry or endeavour to consume long periods of exceptional exercise.

Somehow or another, it's like the Atkins diet, which comparatively supports the muscle to fat ratio's consuming eating just low-carb foods, alongside disposing of foods high in carbs and sugar. Expelling glucose from carbohydrate foods will make the body consume fat for vitality. The significant contrasts between the exemplary keto and the Atkins diet are the previous underlines healthier keto fats, less generally speaking protein and no handled meat, (for example, bacon) while having more research to back up its adequacy.

Truth be told, those distinctions with Atkins layout a portion of the mainstream keto diet fantasies, for example, it is another high-protein plan, suggesting any sort of fat and that scarcely any science inquire about backs up the benefits.

BENEFITS OF KETO DIETS

WEIGHT LOSS

Of the numerous benefits of a keto diet, weight misfortune is frequently considered No. 1., as it can regularly be significant and happen rapidly (particularly for the individuals who begin extremely overweight or large). Those following a keto diet "accomplished better long haul body weight and cardiovascular hazard factor the executives when contrasted with people appointed with a regular low-fat diet (for example a confined vitality diet with under 30 per cent of vitality from fat)."

Keto diet can actuate viable weight misfortune alongside improvement in a few cardiovascular hazard parameters.

To some extent, keto diet weight misfortune is a genuine article since high-fat, low-carb diets can both assistance lessen craving and lift weight misfortune through their hormonal impacts. As portrayed above, when we eat almost no foods that supply us with carbohydrates, we discharge fewer insulin. With lower insulin levels, the body did not store additional vitality as fat for some time in the future and rather can venture into existing fat stores for vitality.

Keto diets are very high in healthy fats, and protein likewise will, in general, be very filling, which can help lessen gorging of void calories, desserts and low-quality nourishments. For the vast majority eating a healthy low-carb diet, it's easy to expend a fitting measure of calories, yet not very many, since things like sugary drinks, Cookies, bread, grains, frozen yoghurt or different desserts and lunchrooms are beyond reach.

Frequently brought about by lymph hub evacuation or harm because of the malignant growth treatment, lymphedema happens on the grounds that there's a blockage in the lymphatic framework and results in the expanding in leg or arm.

DECREASE RISK FOR TYPE 2 DIABETES

This procedure of consuming fat gives a greater number of benefits than just helping us to shed additional weight — it likewise helps control the arrival of hormones like insulin, which assumes a job being developed of diabetes and other health issues. At the point when we eat carbohydrates, insulin is discharged as a response to raised blood glucose (an expansion in sugar coursing in our blood) and insulin levels rise. Insulin is a "capacity hormone" that signals cells to store however much accessible vitality as could reasonably be expected, at first as glycogen (otherwise known as stored carbohydrates in our muscles) and afterwards as muscle versus fat.

The keto diet works by wiping out carbohydrates from your day by day admission and keeping the body's carbohydrate stores practically vacant, in this way keeping an excess of insulin from being discharged following food utilization and making ordinary glucose levels. This can help turn around "insulin obstruction," which is the basic issue adding to diabetes side effects. In contemplates, low-carb diets have indicated benefits for improving circulatory strain, postprandial glycemia and insulin emission.

LESSEN RISK OF HEART DISEASE

The keto diet can lessen the danger of coronary illness markers, including elevated cholesterol and triglycerides. Actually, the keto diet is probably not going to contrarily affect your cholesterol levels, notwithstanding being so high in fat. Additionally, it's fit for lowering cardiovascular infection hazard factors, particularly in the individuals who are fat.

HELP PROTECT AGAINST CANCER

Keto diets may "starve" malignancy cells. An exceptionally handled, master fiery, low-supplement foods can take care of disease cells, making them multiply. What's the association between high-sugar utilization and malignant growth? The ordinary cells found in our bodies can utilize fat for vitality, yet it's accepted that malignant growth cells can't metabolically move to utilize fat as opposed to glucose.

The ketogenic diet is a viable treatment for disease and different genuine health issues.

In this way, a keto diet that kills overabundance refined sugar and other Prepared carbohydrates might be successful in diminishing or battling the disease. It is anything but a fortunate event that probably the best disease battling foods are on the keto diet food list.

BATTLE BRAIN DISEASE AND NEUROLOGICAL DISORDERS

Ketogenic diets have likewise been utilized as normal solutions for a treat, and even assistance turn around neurological scatters and subjective disabilities, including epilepsy, Alzheimer's side effects, hyper misery and uneasiness.

Cutting off glucose levels with a low-carb diet makes your body produce ketones for fuel. This change can assist with turning around neurological clutters and psychological debilitation, including inciting seizure control. The cerebrum can utilize this elective wellspring of vitality rather than the phone vitality pathways that aren't working ordinarily in patients with mind issue.

A related clinical diet for sedate safe epilepsy is known as the medium-chain triglyceride ketogenic diet, in which MCT oil is broadly utilized in light of the fact that it's more ketogenic than long-chain triglycerides.

The report proceeds to state that while these different ailments are obviously unique in relation to one another, the ketogenic diet gives off an impression of being so viable for neurological issues as a result of its "neuroprotective impact" — as the keto seems to address variations from the norm in cell vitality utilization, which is a typical trademark in numerous neurological issue.

A keto diet could slow ailment movement for the two ALS and Huntington's infections. Actually, more than one creature study has found a potential benefit of the low-carb, high-fat diet or discontinuous fasting in postponing weight misfortune, overseeing glucose and shielding neurons from injury.

Strikingly, it's likewise been appeared to slow malady movement in mouse models of the two ALS and Huntington's infections.

The ketogenic diet can likewise assist patients with schizophrenia to standardize the pathophysiological forms that are causing manifestations like daydreams, mental trips, absence of limitation and unusual conduct. The keto diet leads to raised groupings of kynurenic corrosive (KYNA) in the hippocampus and striatum, which advances neuroactive action.
Despite the fact that the specific job of the keto diet in mental and cerebrum issue is hazy, there has been proof of its adequacy in patients with schizophrenia. What's more, for sure, it attempts to invert numerous conditions that create as a symptom of traditional meds for cerebrum issue, similar to weight gain, type 2 diabetes and cardiovascular dangers. More research is expected to comprehend the job of the ketogenic diet in treating or improving schizophrenia, as the ebb and flow accessible examinations are either creature studies or contextual analyses. However, the benefits of a low carbohydrate, high-fat diet in nervous system science is promising.

LIVE LONGER

There's even proof that a low-carb, high-fat routine (as the keto diet may be) encourages you to live more, contrasted with a low-fat diet.

Indeed, immersed fat admission had a backwards relationship with the hazard for experiencing a stroke, which means the more soaked fat somebody is regularly expending, the more insurance against having a stroke they appeared to have.

The keto diet additionally seems to help incite autophagy, which helps clear harmed cells from the body, including senescent cells that fill no practical need yet at the same time, wait inside tissues and organs. In creature examines when rodents are put on the ketogenic diet, autophagic pathways are made that lessen cerebrum injury during and after seizures.

Truth be told, prompting autophagy is presently a famous biohacking procedure for helping expel indications of maturing ineffectively, and keto is one approach to arrive.

A calorie is essentially a method for estimating vitality. The specialized definition is that it is the measure of vitality expected to raise the temperature of one gram of water by one-degree Celsius. For the human body, calories are the vitality the body uses to live, think, breath, and make your heartbeat.

You need a specific number of calories every day to just endure. Indeed, even without moving, your heart is as yet thumping, you need to inhale, your cerebrum needs to work.

This fundamental number of calories you need is called your basal metabolic rate (BMR). It is impacted by your age, sexual orientation, hereditary qualities, body size, body structure and diet. Notwithstanding your BMR, you need extra calories to help your everyday exercises, assimilation, and exercise.

As clarified, a high carb diet diminishes your BMR while a low carb diet, similar to the keto diet builds your BMR. By expanding your BMR, you increment the basic number of calories your body will consume consistently.

If you are keen on knowing what number of calories you need altogether, there are numerous approaches to make sense of this. Metabolic testing is the most precise yet costs cash.

In the event that you are figuring it yourself, the Mifflin St. Jeor condition has been seen as the most precise. It considers sexual orientation, age, and physical action.

Calorie checking isn't really required on keto, yet it can help. It might be particularly helpful when you are simply beginning or in the event that you have arrived at a level. Monitoring what you eat can assist you with getting mindful of what foods work best for you.

Following can assist you with learning segment control and distinguish foods that are high in carbohydrates. It can assist you in making sense of what isn't working. Keeping food records is the same than recording exercise progress or making a monetary spending plan. You can't make changes or improvements without information. The expanded mindfulness can be useful.

In any case, if you will likely lose weight, rather than following each calorie, centre around great food that will advance the arrival of craving smothering hormones to diminish appetite and increment fulfilment. Having a meal arrangement or meal Prepping on a week by week premise will help you right now.

Ensure you have some helpful keto food accessible. Avocados, eggs, coconut oil, MCT oil, verdant greens and other low carb veggies are only a couple of staples that are incredible to keep close by.

Evade foods (even keto inviting ones) that are easy to gorge and high in calories, similar to nuts or cheddar.

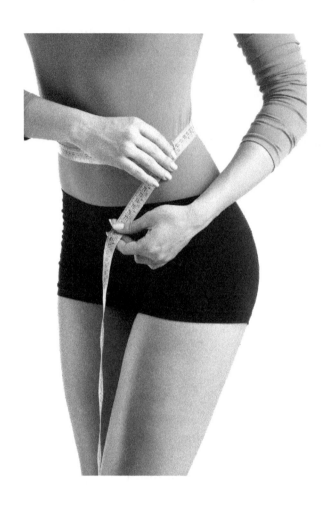

Foods that are edible for you on Ketogenic Diet

Here is a rundown of all the low-carb foods that are proper to eat when you're following keto.

- Fish and seafood

- Low-carb veggies

- Cheese

- Avocados

- poultry

- Eggs

- Nuts, seeds and healthful oils

- Plain Greek yoghurt and curds

- Berries

- Unsweetened espresso and tea

- Dark chocolate and cocoa powder

Fish and Seafood

Fish is plentiful in B nutrients, potassium and selenium; it's additionally protein-rich and sans carb. Salmon, tuna fish, sardines with mackerel, tuna fish and other greasy fish brag high levels of omega-3-fats, which was found to lower glucose levels and increment insulin affectability. Mean to expend at any rate two 3-ounce servings of the greasy fish week after week.

Low-Carb Veggies

Non-starchy vegetables, or non-glucose are low in calories and carbs, however high in numerous supplements, including nutrient C and a few minerals. They likewise contain cancer prevention agents that help secure against cell-harming free radicals. Focus on nonstarchy vegetables with under 8 g of net carbs per cup. Net carbs are Total carbohydrates less fibre. Broccoli, cauliflower, green beans, chime peppers, zucchini and spinach, fit the bill.

Cheddar

Cheddar has zero carbohydrates and is high in fat, making it an extraordinary fit for the ketogenic diet. It's additionally wealthy in protein and calcium. Be that as it may, a 1-ounce cut of cheddar conveys around 30 per cent of the day by day esteem for soaked fat, so in case you're stressed over coronary illness consider partitions while noshing on cheddar.

Plain Greek Yogurt and Cottage Cheese

Yoghurt and curds are high in protein and calcium-rich. Five ounces of plain Greek yoghurt gives only 5 g of carbohydrates and 12 grams of protein. A similar measure of curds additionally has 5 grams of carbohydrates with 18 grams of protein. Studies have indicated that both calcium and protein can diminish craving and advance Totality. Higher-fat yoghurts and curds help keep you full for more, and full-fat items would be a piece of the ketogenic diet.

Avocados

Pick heart-healthy fats like avocados, which are high in monounsaturated fat and potassium. Numerous mineral Americans are deficient. Half medium of avocado contains 9 grams of the Total carbohydrates, 7 grams of which are fibre. Swapping creature fats for plant fats like avocados can help improve cholesterol and triglyceride levels.

Meat and Diary or Poultry.

Meat is an essential source of lean protein and is viewed as a staple on the ketogenic diet. Crisp meat and poultry contain no carbohydrates and are plentiful in B nutrients and a few minerals, including potassium, selenium and zinc. While Prepared meats, similar to bacon and hotdog, are allowed on keto, they aren't the best for your heart and may raise your danger of particular kinds of malignant growth in the event that you eat excessively. Pick chicken, fish and hamburger all the more regularly and point of confinement Prepared meats.

Eggs

Poultry Eggs are high in protein, B nutrients, minerals and cell reinforcements. 2 eggs contain zero carbohydrates and 12 g of protein. Eggs appeared to trigger hormones that expansion sentiments of Totality and keep glucose levels stable, and they likewise contain cell reinforcements, for example, lutein and zeaxanthin, which help ensure eye health.

Nuts, Seeds and Healthy Oils

Nuts and seeds are brimming with healthy polyunsaturated and monounsaturated fats, fibre and protein. They likewise are low in net carbs. Olive oil & coconut oil are the major two oils prescribed on the keto diet. Olive oil is high in oleic corrosive and is related to a lower danger of coronary illness. Coconut oil is high in immersed fat yet contains medium-chain triglycerides (MCTs), which can build ketone creation. MCTs may increment metabolic rate and advance the loss of weight and paunch fat as well. Measure divide sizes while devouring any sort of healthy fat.

Carb means 1 oz. (28 g) of nuts and seeds (net carbohydrate approaches Total carbs short fibre):

- Almonds: 3 g of net carbs (6 g of Total carbs)

- Brazil nuts: 1 g of net carbs (3 g of Total carbs)

- Cashews: 8 g of net carbs (9 g of the Total carbohydrates)

- Macadamia nuts: 2 g of net carbs (4 g of the Total carbs)

- Pecans: 1 g of net carbs (4 g of the Total carbs)

- The Pistachios: 5 g of net carbs (8 g of the Total carbs)

- The walnuts: 2 g net carbs (4 g Total carbs)

- The Chia seeds: 2 g of net carbs (12 g of the Total carbs)

- Flaxseeds: 0 g of net carbs (8 g of the Total carbs)

- The Pumpkin seeds: 2 g of net carbs (4 g of the Total carbs)

- Sesame seeds: 4 g of net carbs (7 g of the Total carbs)

Berries

Berries are wealthy in cancer prevention agents that decrease irritation and secure against ailment. Berries are low in carbohydrates and high in fibre.

Carb means 1/2 cup of certain berries:

- Blackberries: 3 g of net carbs (7 g of the Total carbs)

- Blueberries: 9 g of net carbs (11 g of the Total carbs)

- Raspberries: 3 g of net carbs (7 g of the Total carbs)

- Strawberries: 3 g of net carbs (6 g of the Total carbs)

Unsweetened Coffee and Tea

Plain espresso and tea contain zero grams of carbohydrates, fat or protein, so they are An OK on the keto diet. Studies show espresso lowers the danger of cardiovascular illness and type 2 diabetes. Tea is wealthy in cell reinforcements and has less caffeine than espresso; drinking tea may decrease the danger of coronary failure and stroke, help with weight misfortune and lift your safe framework.

Dim Chocolate and Cocoa Powder

Check the mark on these, as the measure of carbs relies upon the sort and the amount you devour. Cocoa has been known as a "superfruit" in light of the fact that it is wealthy in cancer prevention agents, and dim chocolate contains flavanols, which may diminish the danger of coronary illness by lowering circulatory strain and keeping supply routes healthy.

The ketogenic diet is tied in with accomplishing ketosis, a metabolic express that consumes fat for fuel, rather than carbohydrates or protein. To stay in that increased fat-burning state, you have to restrict your carb admission to 5-10% of your Total calories. For most ladies, that means around 25-40 grams of carbs every day (about the sum in a solitary English biscuit, or one glass of organic product juice)— which is the reason followers of the diet should be so cautious about what they eat, yet what they drink as well. To assist you with picking your tastes admirably, here's a rundown of seven keto-accommodating drinks that will make it somewhat simpler to meet your carb top.

The major Drinks You Can Enjoy on the Keto Diet

Water with lemon or lime

Still or starting zero-calorie, zero-carb water is continually going to be a dieter's best decision. Be that as it may, feel free to include a press of crisp lemon or lime to your glass. The sharp squeezes have an insignificant measure of carbs. Likewise, drinking water before meals has been demonstrated to be a successful method to help check hunger.

Diet pop and other diet refreshments

Most diet soft drinks and refreshments improved with sugar substitutes have zero grams of carbs. Some keto idealists may guarantee sugar subs are not really keto-accommodating, on the grounds that they accept the sweet stuff builds longings for carbs. In any case, there is no proof to propose utilizing without carb sugar substitutes will meddle with your weight-misfortune endeavours. (Likewise, many bundled keto snacks and foods made with sans carb sugars really make it simpler to adhere to a keto way of life longer, so you can lose weight and keep it off.)

While choosing a diet drink, check the Nutrition Facts board to ensure it contains under 5 g Total sugars or 20-calories from carbs. Obviously, you'll have to include any carbohydrates in these drinks against your designated every day carb spending plan.

Remember that when in doubt, diet drinks that are clear have less sketchy ingredients. There are likewise diet drinks, as Zevia, that are improved with all-characteristic stevia.

Espresso and tea (with cream, coconut oil, or margarine)

If you like a spot of margarine whipped into your morning cup of Joe, you'll be glad to discover that impenetrable espresso is for sure keto-accommodating. At the point when you mix fat like margarine or coconut oil or overwhelming cream into your espresso or tea, you do not include carbs.

If you incline toward a progressively customary mug of espresso or tea, you'll have to drink it either with sugar substitutesn or plainly) and with next to no milk since milk contributes some carbs.

The Bovine's milk.

If plaaced on a keto diet, you may drink some milk without disturbing ketosis. For example, A ½ cup of milk has 6 grams of carbs (24 calories) while giving a lot of protein (4 grams), and genuinely necessary supplements like calcium, magnesium, potassium, and nutrient D.

Almond milk

Unsweetened almond milk has around 30 calories for every 8-ounce serving and no sugar, making it an extraordinary choice for those following a keto way of life. Search for brands that are braced with calcium and nutrients An and D.

Keto smoothies

While numerous smoothies are overly sugary gratitude to the foods grown from the ground base, a brisk Google search of "keto smoothie" or "low-carb smoothie" will return a huge number of recipes. The ideal approach to keep carbs low and taste and fulfilment high is to make your smoothie base with fats like nut margarine, avocado, or coconut oil. At that point include some low-carb veggies like verdant greens, cucumbers, celery or beets, and littler measures of fruits like berries, apples or pears. If you need fluid, use ice, water or unsweetened almond milk.

KETO CHAFFLES

What is Chaffee?

A shuffle is a keto waffle. It's known as a chaffle in light of the fact that one of its essential ingredients is destroyed cheddar, thus the CHAffle rather than Waffle, on the grounds that chaffles are cheddar waffles. Adorable right?

Waffles are typically made of a flour-based player. However, a chaffle is sans flour! Rather, chaffless are made of eggs and cheddar. I realize it sounds odd. However, it really works! What's more, dieters wherever are going insane for this new low-carb waffle hack.

Chaffless is an extraordinary path for those on the keto diet to get their waffle fix. They're additionally an incredible method to eat fewer carbs while as yet eating what you need! Regardless of whether it is a changed adaptation. There are additionally unlimited mixes for what you can add to it and how you can spruce up and use chaffless.

The basic formula for a chaffle contains cheddar, almond flour, and an egg. You combine the ingredients in a bowl and pour it on your waffle producer. Waffle creators are most likely on the ascent right now after this chaffle formula detonated a day or two ago prior. I was somewhat doubtful from the outset thinking there was no chance this would turn out in the wake of combining everything and pouring the hitter on the waffle. I was expecting one enormous major chaos. Try to shower the waffle producer truly well. The waffle ended up extraordinary, and it was firm outwardly and delicate in the centre.

Step by step instructions to make chaffles

The main bit of kitchen hardware you have to make these keto chaffles is a waffle producer. I've made chaffles effectively in an ordinary size Belgian waffle producer. What's more, I've made littler size chaffles in a small waffle creator. I like the littler size better for chaffle sandwiches.

It appears as though individuals are having the most achievement utilizing this Dash Mini Waffle Iron. It is the ideal size to Cook them rapidly. Also, the littler size aldes the chaffles fresh up perfectly.

My main tip for making crispier chaffles is to utilize a smaller than usual waffle creator like the Dash. I believe that this small scale waffle creator has the best volume to surface territory proportion to give you the crispiest outcomes.

Another tip is to ensure you Cook the chaffles sufficiently long. For me, it takes around 4 minutes for each chaffle to get brilliant dark colored. They may be somewhat delicate when you first expel them from the waffle creator, yet they will fresh up additional as they cool.

A third tip is to sprinkle some additional cheddar on the chaffle hitter part of the way through Cooking. The cheddar will liquefy and fresh up to make the chaffles extra firm.

You can likewise freeze chaffles. One extraordinary approach to meal Prep is to make a major bunch of chaffles and freeze them to eat later.

To freeze chaffles, freeze them on a Preparing sheet in a solitary layer (so they don't stay together). When they are solidified, place them in a cooler sack with a bit of material paper between each.

In the event that you don't have the cooler space to fit an entire heating sheet, you can freeze them in a cooler sack with a bit of material paper isolating them.

To serve, you can warm them in the microwave for 2-3 minutes. On the off chance that you have additional time, you can warm in a 350F stove or air fryer for crispier outcomes.

You can add a wide range of flavourings to plain chaffle hitter to make new kinds of chaffles.

- Try exploring different avenues regarding various types of cheddar. Cheddar is the first flavour, yet in addition use Monterrey Jack, Colby, mozzarella cheddar, and so on. You could even consolidate two various types of cheddar for included flavour — like a blend of mozzarella and Parmesan for a seasoned Italian Chaffle.

- Add flavours, for example, garlic powder, Italian flavouring, Everything except the Bagel flavouring, or arranged herbs.

- Experiment with including keto-accommodating fruits and vegetables to your chaffle hitter. Think little solidified blueberries, or finely hacked peppers and onions.

- For much lighter chaffles, you can include a teaspoon of coconut flour or a tablespoon of almond flour to the egg blend. For a definitive fluffiest chaffles, include 1/4 tsp Preparing powder and a spot of salt.

- For sweet chaffles, you can include a tablespoon of keto-accommodating sugars like Confectioner's Swerve or Lakanto maple syrup. Remember Lily's chocolate chips!

INGREDIENTS

- 1 egg

- 1/2 cup cheddar, destroyed

- 1 tbsp almond flour (discretionary, see formula notes for different alternatives)

Directions

1. Preheat the waffle creator as indicated by maker guidelines.

2. In a little blending bowl, combine egg and cheddar. Mix until all around consolidated.

3. Optionally, include the almond flour. See formula notes for more thoughts.

4. If utilizing a smaller than usual waffle producer, pour one portion of the waffle hitter into the waffle creator.

5. Cook for 3-4 minutes or until it arrives at wanted doneness. Rehash with the second 50% of the hitter.

NOTES

- See the formula varieties in the post above for thoughts regarding making lighter or fluffier waffles. You can make extremely scrumptious chaffles with simply the cheddar and egg.

- But, if you need lighter and fluffier chaffles, you can include either 1 teaspoonful of coconut flour and or 1 tablespoonful of the almond flour to the batter.

- You can likewise season your chaffle player with a spot of garlic powder, dried herbs, Italian flavouring, or Everything Bagel flavouring.

- If you are utilizing a bigger size waffle producer, you might have the option to Cook the entire measure of hitter in one waffle. This will change with the size of your machine.

The Best Flours to be taken on a Keto Diet

When beginning a keto diet, numerous individuals need to re-make their most loved non-keto foods to help with consistency on a keto diet. Numerous foods individuals look to re-make are bread, buns, biscuits, Cookies, brownies, cakes, tortillas, and numerous other flour-based foods.

In case you're fresh out of the plastic new to keto, below are a rundown of our preferred flours to use on a keto diet.

The Best Flours to to be taken on a Keto Diet

Coconut Flour is exceptionally high in fibre and low in carbohydrates, so it is immaculate to use in Prepared merchandise, for example, bread and desserts. Since it is high in fibre it typically just requires around 1/4 the sum if subbing instead of ordinary flour or the almond flour.

The Almond Flour is high in fat, and low in carbs, and moderate in protein. It is denser than coconut flour and is typically a 1:1 substitute for the standard flour, dissimilar to the coconut flour.

Psyllium Husk Flour is a flour that I had never utilized I begun to follow a ketogenic diet. It's high in fibre and is generally utilized in bread and move recipes.

Ground Flax Seed is high in fibre and fat and is pressed loaded with ALA Omega 3 fatties' acids.

Ground Chia Seeds are high in protein and fibre and have 0g net carbs per serving. They are extraordinary for utilizing in Prepared merchandise, yet I like utilizing ground chia for smoothies since it tends to not stick within the blender as customary chia seeds do.

Ground Sunflower Seeds. I've seen a great deal of pre-made Preparing blends utilize this as their flour of decision. They make for extremely chewy Cookies and brownies!

Cricket Flour. If you are feeling bold? Cricket flour has 2g fat, 1g carb and 7g protein per 10g serving.

Oat Fiber. With 3g of carbs all originating from fibre, this flour is flawless to add to Prepared great without the dread of spiking your glucose.

Wheat flour contains gluten—the protein that reinforces and ties mixture in Preparing. Along these lines, when heating with wheat-free flours, you will ordinarily need to source elective restricting specialists. Allude to What are the options to thickener or guar gum? For proposals.

In case you're following particular wheat-free or gluten-free formula it will have been deliberately detailed to get the ideal outcome utilizing the flour substitutes recorded. In the event that you are subbing other elective flours to those recorded you should know that you may get a disappointment, so don't do it just because if Cooking for a significant event.

A decent tip in the event that you do need to substitute a gluten-free flour is to utilize a flour of comparable properties and weight. For instance, custard flour may substitute alright for arrowroot flour.

The flours recorded below are options in contrast to wheat, grain, or rye flours. Anyway, it is imperative to know that there is no accurate substitute for gluten-containing flour, and recipes made with wheat and gluten-free elective flours will be not quite the same as those containing wheat or gluten.

It's in every case best to store flours in hermetically sealed compartments in a dull, cool spot to maintain a strategic distance from them turning smelly. It's ideal to utilize them at room temperature; however, so measure out what you need and let them warm up somewhat.

Amaranth flour

Amaranth flour is produced using the seed of the Amaranth plant, which is a verdant vegetable. Amaranth seeds are high in protein, which makes a nutritious flour for Preparing—elective names: African spinach, Chinese spinach, Indian spinach, elephants ear.

Wheat-free Gluten-free

Arrowroot flour

Arrowroot flour is ground from the foundation of the plant and is extremely valuable for thickening recipes. It is boring, and the fine powder turns out to be clear when it is Cooked, which makes it perfect for clear thickening sauces.

Wheat-free Gluten-free

Banana flour

It is produced using unripe green bananas that are dried and processed to make a flour that has a grain-like taste rather than a banana taste. Can be used for all Cooking and heating, or as a thickener for soups and sauces. Utilize 25% less banana flour than is proposed for flour in recipes.

Wheat-free Gluten-free

Grain flour

The grain just contains a modest quantity of gluten, so is once in a while used to make bread, except for unleavened bread. It has a somewhat nutty flavour and can be utilized to thicken or enhance soups or stews. Mixed with other elective flours, it is additionally genuinely flexible for cakes, bread rolls, baked good, dumplings and so on.

Wheat-free Gluten-free

Darker rice flour

Darker rice flour is heavier than its family member, white rice flour. It is processed from unpolished dark coloured rice, so it has a higher nutritional incentive than white, and as it contains the wheat of the darker rice, it has a higher fibre content. This additionally implies it has an observable surface, somewhat grainy.

It has a nutty taste, which sometimes turn out in recipes relying upon different ingredients, and the surface will likewise add to a heavier item than recipes made with white rice flour. It is a rare occurrence utilized Totally all alone due to its heavier nature.

Mass purchasing isn't suggested as it is better utilized when crisp, store in an impenetrable compartment.

Wheat-free Gluten-free

Buckwheat flour

Buckwheat flour isn't, regardless of its name a type of wheat, buckwheat is really identified with rhubarb. The little seeds of the plant are ground to make flour.

It has a solid nutty taste so isn't commonly utilized all alone in a formula, as the flavour of the completed item can be exceptionally overwhelming, and somewhat harsh—elective names: beech wheat, kasha, Saracen corn.

Wheat-free Gluten-free

Chia flour

Produced using ground chia seeds. Profoundly nutritious, chia seeds have been marked a "superfood" containing Omega 3, fibre, calcium and protein, all stuffed into little seeds.

Otherwise called "nature's rocket fuel" the same number of sportspeople and superathletes, for example, the Tarahumara use it for upgraded vitality levels during occasions.

On the off chance that chia flour isn't promptly accessible, at that point put chia seeds in a processor and whizz up a few. Whenever utilized in Preparing, fluid levels and heating time may be expanded marginally.

Wheat-free Gluten-free

Chickpea flour (otherwise called gram or garbanzo flour)

This is ground from chickpeas and has a solid marginally nutty taste. It isn't commonly utilized all alone.

Wheat-free Gluten-free

Coconut flour

Produced using dried, defatted coconut meat this flour is high in fibre with a light coconut enhance. Commonly extra fluid will be required in a formula that utilizes coconut flour.

Wheat-free Gluten-free

Coffee Flour

Produced using the disposed of espresso cherry natural product this is a nutritious flour that doesn't taste of espresso. The natural espresso product is processed into a flour that is high in fibre, and low in fat, which also has more iron than most grains, and is low in caffeine, and has more potassium than bananas.

Wheat-free Gluten-free

Cornflour

Cornflour is processed from corn into a fine, white powder, and is utilized for thickening recipes and sauces. It has a dull taste, and in this manner is utilized related to different ingredients that will bestow flavour to the formula.

It additionally works very well when blended in with different flours, for instance, when making fine players for tempura.

A few sorts of cornflour are processed from wheat; however, are marked wheaten cornflour.

Elective name: cornstarch.

Wheat-free Gluten-free

Cornmeal

Ground from corn. Heavier than cornflour, not for the most part compatible in recipes.

Wheat-free Gluten-free

Hemp flour

Produced using ground hemp seeds it has a gentle, nutty flavour.

Wheat-free Gluten-free

Lupin flour

Produced using a vegetable in a similar plant family as peanuts. It is increasingly high in protein and fibre, low in fat yet conveys a similar protein that causes hypersensitive responses/hypersensitivity to nut or vegetables, which makes it unsatisfactory for individuals with nut or vegetable sensitivities for example soybeans.

Wheat-free Gluten-free

Maize flour

Ground from corn. Heavier than cornflour, not for the most part exchangeable in recipes.

Wheat-free Gluten-free

Millet flour

Originates from the grass family, and is utilized as an oat in numerous African and Asian nations. It may be used to thicken soups and make level bread and frying pancakes. Since it comes up short on any type of gluten, it's not fit to numerous sorts of Preparing.

Wheat-free Gluten-free

Oat flour

Ground from oats care should be taken to guarantee that it is sourced from a non-wheat tainting process. Likewise contains avenin, which is a protein like gluten, so even guaranteed gluten-free oats may not be appropriate for all celiacs.

Ingests fluids more than numerous flours, so may need to build the fluid substance of any formula it is added to. Promptly substitutes into many cakes and treat recipes. Oat flour goes foul rapidly, either purchase modest quantities or use rapidly, store it in the ice chest/cooler, or make your own utilizing a food processor.

Wheat-free Gluten-free

Potato flour

This flour ought not to be mistaken for potato starch flour. Potato flour has a solid potato season and is a substantial flour, so a little goes far. Mass purchasing isn't suggested except if you are utilizing it all the time for an assortment of recipes as it doesn't have a long time span of usability.

Wheat-free Gluten-free

Potato starch flour

This is a fine white flour produced using potatoes and has a light potato season which is imperceptible when utilized in recipes. It's one of only a handful, not many elective flours that keeps very much gave it is stored in a sealed shut container, and someplace cool and dim.

Wheat-free Gluten-free

Quinoa flour (articulated 'sharp wa')

Quinoa is identified with the plant group of spinach and beets. It has been utilized for more than 5,000 years as a grain, and the Incas considered it the mother seed. Quinoa gives a decent wellspring of vegetable protein, and it is the seeds of the quinoa plant that are ground to make flour.

Wheat-free Gluten-free

Rye flour

Rye flour is an emphatically seasoned flour, dull in shading. Bread made with rye flour is denser than those made with wheat, for instance, pumpernickel which is for all intents and purposes dark. Rye flour has a low gluten content, yet it can likewise be utilized for recipes, for example, hotcakes and biscuits.

Wheat-free Gluten-free

Sorghum flour

Ground from sorghum grain, which is like millet. The flour is utilized to make porridge or level unleavened bread. It is a significant staple in Africa and India.

This flour stores well under typical temperatures.

Wheat-free Gluten-free

Soya flour

Soya flour is a type of flour that is high protein flour with a nutty taste. It isn't commonly utilized all alone in recipes; however, when joined with different flours is fruitful as an elective flour. Can be utilized to thicken recipes or included as a flavour enhancer.

It should be painstakingly stored as it is a high-fat flour and can go rank if not stored appropriately. A cool, dim condition is prescribed and can even be stored in the fridge.

Wheat-free Gluten-free

Custard flour

Custard flour is produced using the base of the cassava plant when ground it appears as a light, delicate, fine white flour. Custard flour adds chewiness to heating and is a decent thickener. Custard flour is a phenomenal expansion to any wheat-free kitchen. It's a genuinely strong flour, so putting away at room temperature is no issue.

Wheat-free Gluten-free

Teff flour

Teff originates from the grass family and is a small oat grain local to northern Africa. It is currently finding a speciality in the health food advertising on the grounds that it is nutritious.

Wheat-free Gluten-free

White rice flour

This flour is processed from cleaned white rice, so it is extremely dull in taste, and not especially nutritious. White rice flour is perfect for recipes that require a light surface; for instance, our herby dumplings. It very well may be utilized all alone for an assortment of recipes and has a sensible time span of usability, as long as it is stored in an impenetrable compartment to evade it retaining dampness from the air.

Wheat-free Gluten-free

There are numerous flours you don't use in wheat-free Cooking, more subtleties...

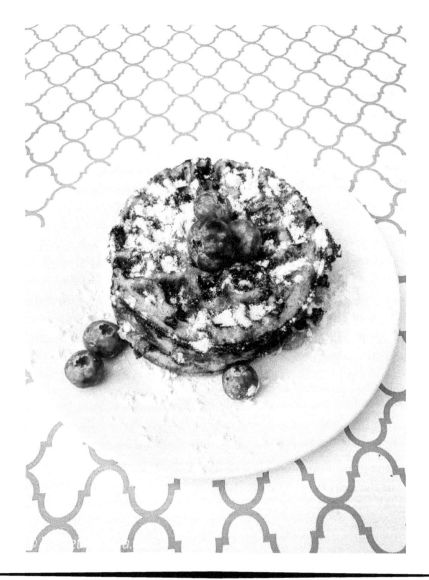

15 RECIPES FOR BASIC FLAVORED CHAFFLES

Nutty spread Cup Chaffles

Yield: 1 PEANUT BUTTER CUP CHAFFLE

Prep time: 10 MINUTES

Cook time: 6 MINUTES

Total time: 16 MINUTES

Thick chocolate chaffles spread with a thick layer of smooth, sweet, nutty spread!

Ingredients

For the chaffle:

♣ 1 huge egg

♣ 2 tablespoons cocoa powder

♣ 1 tablespoon sugar

♣ 1 tablespoon sugar freechocolate chips

♣ 1/4 teaspoon coffee powder

♣ 1/2 cup finely destroyed mozzarella

For the nutty spread filling:

♣ 3 tablespoons smooth nutty spread

♣ 2 tablespoons powdered sugar

♣ 1 tablespoon spread, mellowed

Directions

To make the chaffles:

1. Plug in the waffle iron to preheat.

2. Whisk together the egg, cocoa powder, sugar, chocolate slashes, and coffee powder. Mix in the mozzarella.

3. Add portion of the player to the waffle creator and Cook for 3 minutes. Rehash with outstanding player.

To make the nutty spread filling:

1. Add the entirety of the ingredients to a little bowl and mix together with a fork until smooth and velvety.

To amass:

1. Let waffles cool before spreading with the nutty spread and shutting to shape a sandwich.

Notes

If you don't mind note that I've deducted sugar alcohols from this formula as erythritol, for the most part, has no impact on glucose. In the event that you include sugar alcohols in your carb check, you'll need to compute this yourself.
Nutrition Information:

YIELD: 4 SERVING SIZE: 1/4 of waffle

Sum Per Serving: CALORIES: 210TOTAL FAT: 15gSATURATED FAT: 5gTRANS FAT: 0gUNSATURATED FAT: 8gCHOLESTEROL: 61mgSODIUM: 208mgCARBOHYDRATES: 4gNET CARBOHYDRATES: 3gFIBER: 1gSUGAR: 2gPROTEIN: 8g

Large Mac Chaffle

Yield: 1 BIG MAC

Prep time: 10 MINUTES

Cook time: 10 MINUTES

Total time: 20 MINUTES

These cheeseburger chaffles pose a flavour like my preferred cheap food burger, directly down to the mystery ingredient! Don't hesitate to twofold or even fourfold this formula in case you're taking care of multiple!

Ingredients

For the cheeseburgers:

♣ 1/3 pound ground hamburger

♣ 1/2 teaspoon garlic salt

♣ 2 cuts American cheddar

For the Chaffles:

♣ 1 enormous egg

♣ 1/2 cup finely destroyed mozzarella

♣ 1/4 teaspoon garlic salt

For the Big Mac Sauce:

♣ 2 teaspoons mayonnaise

♣ 1 teaspoon ketchup

♣ 1 teaspoon dill pickle relish

♣ splash vinegar, to taste

To collect:

♣ 2 tablespoons destroyed lettuce

♣ 3-4 dill pickles

♣ 2 teaspoons minced onion

Guidelines

- To make the burgers:

- Warmth an iron over medium-high warmth.

- Partition the ground hamburger into 2 equivalent measured balls and spot each on the frying pan, at any rate, 6 inches separated.

- Let Cook for 1 moment.

- Utilize a little serving of mixed greens plate to immovably squeeze straight down on the bundles of hamburger to straighten. Sprinkle with garlic salt.

- Cook 2 minutes or until mostly Cooked through. Flip the burgers cautiously and sprinkle with outstanding garlic salt.

- Keep Cooking 2 minutes or until Cooked through.

- Spot one cut of cheddar over every patty and afterwards stack the patties and put aside on a plate. Spread with foil.

- To make the chaffles:

- Warmth the smaller than normal waffle iron and splash with non-stick shower.

- Whisk together the egg, cheddar, and garlic salt until very much consolidated.

- Include half of the egg blend to the waffle iron and Cook for 2-3 minutes. Put in a safe spot and rehash with an outstanding player.

- To make the Big Mac Sauce:

- Whisk together all ingredients.

- To amass burgers:

- Top one chaffle with the stacked burger patties, destroyed lettuce, pickles, and onions.

- Spread the Big Mac sauce over the other chaffle and spot sauce side down over the sandwich.

- Eat right away.

Notes

Don't hesitate to twofold or fourfold this formula.

Nutrition Information:

YIELD: 1 SERVING SIZE: 1

Sum Per Serving: CALORIES: 831TOTAL FAT: 56gSATURATED FAT: 23gTRANS FAT: 2gUNSATURATED FAT: 26g CHOLESTEROL: 382mgSODIUM: 3494mgCARBOHYDRATES: 8gNET CARBOHYDRATES: 6gFIBER: 2gSUGAR: 2gPROTEIN: 65g

Garlic Bread Chaffle

Yield: 2 SERVINGS

Prep time: 5 MINUTES

Cook time: 10 MINUTES

Total time: 15 MINUTES

Gooey garlic bread made in minutes on account of your waffle producer!

Ingredients

♣ 1 huge egg

♣ 1/2 cup finely destroyed mozzarella

♣ 1 teaspoon coconut flour

♣ ¼ teaspoon Preparing powder

♣ ½ teaspoon garlic powder

♣ 1 tablespoon spread, softened

♣ 1/4 teaspoon garlic salt

♣ 2 tablespoons Parmesan

♣ 1 teaspoon minced parsley

Directions

1. Plug in your small waffle iron to preheat. Preheat broiler to 375 degrees.

2. Add the egg, mozzarella, coconut flour, Preparing powder, and garlic powder to a blending bowl and whisk well to join.

3. Pour a portion of the chaffle hitter into the waffle iron and Cook for 3 minutes or until the steam stops. Spot the chaffle on a heating sheet.

4. Repeat with the remaining chaffle hitter.

5. Stir together the margarine and garlic salt and brush over the chaffles.

6. Top the chaffles with the Parmesan.

7. Place the container in the broiler for 5 minutes to liquefy the cheddar.

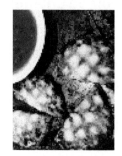

8. Sprinkle with parsley before serving.

Notes

The garlic salt makes these somewhat salty - don't hesitate to swap in crisp minced garlic or garlic powder, in case you're watching salt.

Nutrition Information:

YIELD: 2 servings SERVING SIZE: 1

Sum Per Serving: CALORIES: 186TOTAL FAT: 14gSATURATED FAT: 8gTRANS FAT: 0gUNSATURATED FAT: 5gCHOLESTEROL: 127mgSODIUM: 590mgCARBOHYDRATES: 3gNET CARBOHYDRATES: 2gFIBER: 1gSUGAR: 1gPROTEIN: 10g

Basic Chaffle Recipe

Yield: 2 WAFFLES

Prep time: 1 MINUTE

Cook time: 6 MINUTES

Total time: 7 MINUTES

These chaffles are only two ingredients and Cook in only a couple of moments! Flawless spread with margarine and sugar-free syrup.

Ingredients

♣ 1 enormous egg

♣ 1/2 cup finely destroyed mozzarella

Guidelines

1. Plugin the waffle producer to warm.

2. Break the egg into a little bowl and race with a fork. Add the mozzarella and mix to consolidate.

3. Spray the waffle iron with non-stick shower.

4. Pour a portion of the egg blend into the warmed waffle iron and Cook for 2-3 minutes.

5. Remove waffle cautiously and Cook remaining player.

6. Serve warm with margarine and without sugar syrup.

Notes

Have a go at including a sprinkle of vanilla or run of cinnamon for next-level breakfast chaffles!

Nutrition Information:

YIELD: 1 SERVING SIZE: 2 waffles

Sum Per Serving: CALORIES: 202TOTAL FAT: 13gSATURATED FAT: 6gTRANS FAT: 0gUNSATURATED FAT: 5g CHOLESTEROL: 214mg SODIUM: 364mg CARBOHYDRATES: 3g NET CARBOHYDRATES: 3gFIBER: 0gSUGAR: 1gPROTEIN: 16g

Strawberry Shortcake Chaffle

This low carb and keto benevolent Strawberry Shortcake Chaffle is the ideal dessert to appreciate after dinner!

Prep Time4 minutes

Cook Time12 minutes

Servings3 Chaffles

Ingredients

Strawberry besting Ingredients

• 3 new strawberries

• 1/2 tablespoon granulated swerve

Sweet Chaffle Ingredients

• 1 tablespoon almond flour

• 1/2 cup mozzarella cheddar

• 1 egg

• 1 tablespoon granulated swerve

• 1/4 teaspoon vanilla concentrate

• Keto Whipped Cream

Directions

1. Heat up your waffle creator. If you are utilizing a smaller than usual waffle producer this formula will make 2 chaffles, if utilizing a huge waffle creator, this formula will make 1 enormous sweet chaffle.

2. Rinse and slash up your new strawberries. Spot the strawberries in a little bowl and include 1/2 tablespoon granulated swerve. Blend the strawberries in with the swerve and put in a safe spot.

3. In a bowl blend the almond flour, egg, mozzarella cheddar, granulated swerve and vanilla concentrate.

4. Pour 1/3 of the player into your smaller than usual waffle creator and Cook for 3-4 minutes. At that point Cook another 1/3 of the player and the remainder of the hitter to make 3 keto chaffles.

5. While your second chaffle is Cooking, make your keto whipped cream in the event that you don't have any available.

6. Assemble your Strawberry Shortcake Chaffle by putting whipped cream and strawberries on your sweet chaffle. At that point sprinkle the juice that will likewise be in the bowl with the strawberries on top.

Nutrition

Serving: 1g | Calories: 112kcal | Carbohydrates: 2g| Protein: 7g | Fat: 8g | Saturated Fat: 3g | Cholesterol: 69mg | Sodium: 138mg | Potassium: 53mg | Fiber: 1g | Sugar: 1g | Vitamin A: 205IU | Vitamin C: 7mg | Calcium: 107mg | Iron: 1mg

Course chaffle, Dessert, keto, low carb

Cooking American

Catchphrases Chaffle Recipe, Keto Chaffle, keto chaffle formula, Strawberry Shortcake Chaffle

Keto Blueberry Chaffle

This delectable keto blueberry waffle is in fact called a Keto Chaffle! Furthermore, a kid is it delish! Consummately sweet, with succulent blueberries, these blueberry keto chaffles taste extraordinary and are low carb and keto agreeable.

Prep Time3 minutes

Cook Time15 minutes

Servings5 Chaffles

Hardware

• Dash smaller than expected waffle producer

Ingredients

- 1 cup of mozzarella cheddar

- 2 tablespoons almond flour

- 1 tsp heating powder

- 2 eggs

- 1 tsp cinnamon

- 2 tsp of Swerve

- 3 tablespoon blueberries

Guidelines

1. Heat up your Dash smaller than expected waffle producer.

2. In a blending, bowl include the mozzarella cheddar, almond flour, heating powder, eggs, cinnamon, swerve and blueberries. Blend well, so all the ingredients are combined.

3. Spray your smaller than expected waffle producer with non-stick Cooking shower.

4. Add shortly under 1/4 a cup of blueberry keto waffle player.

5. Close the top and Cook the chaffle for 3-5 minutes. Check it at the 3-minute imprint to check whether it is fresh and darker. In the event that it isn't or it adheres to the highest point of the waffle machine close the cover and Cook for 1-2 minutes longer.

6. Serve with a sprinkle of swerving confectioners' sugar or keto syrup.

Notes

Net carbs - 2g net of carbs per blueberry chaffle

Nutritional facts

Serving: 1g | Calories: 115kcal | Carbohydrates: 5g | Protein: 8g | Fat: 8.5g | Saturated Fat: 4g | Cholesterol: 84mg | Sodium: 165mg | Potassium: 142mg | Fiber: 1g | Sugar: 1g | Vitamin A: 245IU | Vitamin C: 1mg | Calcium: 178mg | Iron: 1mg

Course Breakfast, keto, low carb

Cooking American

Catchphrases Blueberry Keto Chaffle, Blueberry Keto Waffle, Keto Chaffle

Keto Chaffle Garlic Cheesy Bread Sticks

Prep Time: 3 minutes

Cook Time: 7 minutes

Total Time: 10 minutes

Servings: 8 sticks

Calories: 74kcal

Ingredients

- 1 medium egg

- 1/2 cup mozzarella cheddar ground

- 2 tablespoons almond flour

- 1/2 teaspoon garlic powder

- 1/2 teaspoon oregano

- 1/2 teaspoon salt

Besting

- 2 tablespoons spread, unsalted mellowed

- 1/2 teaspoon garlic powder

- 1/4 cup mozzarella cheddar ground

Directions

1. Turn on your waffle creator and daintily oil it (I give it a light shower with olive oil)

2. In a bowl, beat the egg.

3. Add the mozzarella, almond flour, garlic powder, oregano and salt and blend well.

4. Spoon the hitter into your waffle creator (mine is a square twofold waffle, and this blend covers both waffle areas. In the event that you are utilizing a littler waffle creator spoon a large portion of the blend in at once).

5. I spoon my blend into the focal point of my waffle creator and tenderly spread it out towards the edges.

6. Close the cover of the pot and Cook for 5 minutes.

7. Using tongs, expel the Cooked waffles and cut into 4 strips for each waffle.

8. Place the sticks on a plate and pre-heat the flame broil.

9. Mix the margarine with the garlic powder and spread over the sticks.

10. Sprinkle the mozzarella over the sticks and spot under the flame broil for 2-3 minutes until the cheddar has dissolved and percolating.

11. Eat right away! (If we have gobbled this warmed up yet are a lot more pleasant crisply made)

Notes

The net carbohydrates will then be the Total carb check less the fiber tally. Carb tally prohibits sugar alcohols.

Varieties may happen for different reasons, including item accessibility and food Preparation. We make no portrayal or guarantee of the precision of this data.

Nutrition

Serving: 1stick | Calories: 74kcal | Carbohydrates: 0.9g | Protein: 3.4g | Fat: 6.5g | Fiber: 0.2g

Keto Cream Cheese Mini Chaffle Waffles

To begin, here is a straightforward and sweet low-carb/keto waffle formula for your smaller than normal waffle iron, ideal for all you morning sweet tooth's out there! These waffles are somewhat sweet with a trace of coconut and a mess of delightfulness!

All at just ~2 net carb per waffle! Presently you have your reason to eat waffles throughout the day!

Just, all things considered, these won't be 'firm' waffles, yet rather 'gentler' waffles. In case you're searching for fresh, this formula would work better, yet it's not sweet.

For this dish, the uncommon ingredients you would require are Coconut Flour and Swerve/Monkfruit, which can be bought on Amazon or a nearby claim to general fame store. You will likewise require a waffle producer. Utilize the Dash Mini Waffle Maker since it makes the ideal size waffles, yet any waffle creator will do.

Note – If you are Preparing various servings, we will prescribe utilizing 2 Dash Mini Waffle Maker at the same time to decrease the Cooking time.

Prepping Time 3M

Cooking Time 8M

Total Time 11M

Net Carb/Waffle ~2g

Servings 2 Waffles

INGREDIENTS

• 2 tsp Coconut Flour

• 4 tsp Swerve/Monkfruit

• 1/4 tsp Baking Powder

• 1 Egg (room temp)

• 1 oz Cream Cheese (room temp)

• 1/2 tsp Vanilla Extract

Keto Salted Caramel Frappuccino

In the event that you are needing your ordinary frappuccino from Starbucks and are keto/Low Carb, at that point you are going to cherish this Keto Salted Caramel Frappuccino!

Prep Time5 minutes

Cook Time5 minutes

Total Time10 minutes

Servings1

Ingredients

• 1 mug espresso solidified in an ice plate

• 1 mug espresso

• 3 tablespoons overwhelming cream

• 3 tablespoons without sugar caramel syrup

• 5 drops fluid stevia extricate

• tablespoon without sugar caramel sauce sprinkle

Directions

1. In the blender, add the espresso ice 3D squares, espresso, substantial cream, caramel syrup, and stevia.

2. Blend it for 30 seconds, or until smooth.

3. While the drink is mixing, get your premade got cream or whip ready a bunch of keto whipped cream.

4. Place the whipped cream in a cake pack with a star tip.

5. Take your cup and include a twirl of the caramel around within the cup.

6. Pour the Frappuccino blend into the cup and top it with the whipped cream.

Nutrition

Calories: 159kcal | Carbohydrates: 2g | Protein: 1g | Fat: 16g | Saturated Fat: 10g | Cholesterol: 61mg | Sodium: 26mg | Potassium: 232mg | Vitamin A: 660IU | Calcium: 29mg

Catchphrases Keto Salted Caramel Frappuccino

The keto Cheese Chips.

The Keto Cheese Chips made in the Microwave are a delectable and fast Keto nibble. They are likewise ideal for including top of servings of mixed greens!

Prep Time1 minute

Cook Time1 minute

Total Time2 minutes

Servings1

Ingredients

• 3 ounces Sharp Cheddar Cheese Roughly 6 cuts of full-sized cheddar cuts

Directions

1. Line a microwave-safe plate with a bit of material paper.

2. If you are utilizing full-size bits of cheddar, cut your cheddar cut into fourths. If you are using a square of cheddar you have to cut your cheddar here, and in the event that you are utilizing pre-cut cheddar, you can skirt this progression.

3. Arrange the cheddar on the plate, making a point to leave room between the cuts, so they don't run together.
4. Microwave on high for one moment.

5. Remove the material paper from the plate and allow the cheddar to cool.

6. If any of the chips liquefied together, you can cautiously break them separated or simply appreciate a huge chip.

Notes

Nutrition data is dependent on 3 ounces of Sharp Cheddar Cheese, anyway, most cheddar has 0 carbs, so regardless of what cheddar you are utilizing you will at present have a 0 carb cheddar chip.

Nutrition

Calories: 342kcal | Protein: 21g | Fat: 28g | Saturated Fat: 17g | Cholesterol: 89mg | Sodium: 528mg | Potassium: 83mg | Vitamin A: 850IU | Calcium: 613mg | Iron: 0.6mg

Course Appetizer, Snack

Food American

Watchwords cheddar chips, Keto Cheese Chips, Keto Cheese Crackers, Keto Cheese Crisps

Greek Marinated Feta And Olives

A heavenly Mediterranean diet propelled starter or bite, that is likewise low carb, these marinated olives and feta cheddar are ideal for any individual who is searching for an easy delectable formula.

Prep Time5 minutes

Cook Time5 minutes

Cool15 minutes

Servings4

Ingredients

• 1 cup olive oil

• 1/4 teaspoon oregano

• 1/4 teaspoon thyme

• 1/2 teaspoon dried rosemary

• 1 cup kalamata olives

• 1 cup of green olives

• 1/2 pound feta

Guidelines

1. In a little pan heat the oil, oregano, thyme, rosemary together over medium warmth for 5 minutes to inject the oil with the herbs.

2. Set the oil to the side and allow it to cool for 15 minutes.

3. Cut the feta into 1/2 inch shapes.

4. In a medium combining bowl tenderly mix the oil, olives, and feta.

5. Transfer into a sealed shut compartment, and store in the ice chest. You need the olives to marinate for at any rate 20 minutes before you eat them.

6. Serve the olives at room temperature. You should take the olives out a tad before serving them, so the olive oils heat up.

Notes

There are 3g net carbs per serving. 5g carbs - 2g fiber = 3g net carbs.

Nutrition

Calories: 296kcal | Carbohydrates: 5g | Protein: 9g | Fat: 28g | Saturated Fat: 11g | Cholesterol: 50mg | Sodium: 1683mg | Potassium: 64mg | Fiber: 2g | Sugar: 3g | Vitamin A: 505IU | Calcium: 315mg | Iron: 0.7mg

Course Appetizer, Lunch, Snack

Cooking American, Greek

Catchphrases Greek Marinated Olives, Greek olives with feta, Marinated Olives with Feta

Caprese Skewers

Prep Time: 14 minutes

Marinating Time: 3 hours

Total Time: 3 hours 14 minutes

Servings: 14 sticks

Calories: 64kcal

Ingredients

• 14 Mozzarella balls Bocconcini

• 14 cherry tomatoes

- 14 basil leaves

- 7 dark olives cut down the middle

MARINADE

- 3 tablespoons olive oil

- 1 garlic clove hacked

- 1 teaspoon oregano dried

- 1/2 teaspoon salt

- 1/2 teaspoon dark pepper

Directions

1. Mix the marinade in a Ziplock sack (or bowl with cover)

2. Add the tomato and bocconcini (mozzarella balls). Shake well and marinate for at least 3 hours (medium-term is perfect).

3. Assemble the tomatoes, cheddar on a medium estimated toothpick. Include a large portion of olive the top with a leaf of basil.

4. Drizzle any outstanding marinade or pesto to serve.

Notes

Varieties may happen for different reasons, including item accessibility and food Preparation. We make no portrayal or guarantee of the precision of this data.

Nutrition

Serving: 1skewer | Calories: 64kcal | Carbohydrates: 1.1g | Protein: 2.7g | Fat: 5.6g | Fiber: 0.3g

Cauliflower Cheese Jalapeno Soup

Prep Time: 10 minutes

Cook Time: 40 minutes

Total Time: 50 minutes

Servings: 6 servings

Calories: 180kcal

Ingredients

- 1 head cauliflower cut into florets

- 2 tablespoons olive oil

- 1 medium onion stripped and hacked

- 3 cloves garlic stripped and hacked

- 4 jalapeno peppers deseeded and hacked

- 500 ml stock - either vegetable or chicken

- 2 cups cheddar ground

- 1 teaspoon salt

- 1 teaspoon dark pepper

Directions

1. Heat the olive oil in a huge pan on a medium warmth and include the cauliflower florets. Cook for around 5-8 minutes, turning much of the time until marginally brilliant in shading.

2. Add the onion, the garlic and the jalapeno and then Cook for a further 3 minutes.

3. Add stock and bring to the bubble, spread, and stew for around 20 minutes until the cauliflower is delicate.

4. Add the cheddar and season to taste. Cook for around 5 minutes until the cheddar has softened.

5. Remove from the warmth and mix either by utilizing a hand blender or emptying the soup into a blender.

6. Serve, gulp and appreciate!

Notes

Other ground cheddar can be utilized. Attempt a Gruyere.

The Total carbs will now be the Total carb tally less the fibre tally. Carb tally prohibits sugar alcohols.

Varieties may happen for different reasons, including item accessibility and food Preparation. We make no portrayal or guarantee of the exactness of this data.

Nutrition

Serving: 1serving | Calories: 180kcal | Carbohydrates: 6.2g | Protein: 11g | Fat: 13g | Fiber: 2.1g

Mushroom Tarragon Soup

Prep Time: 5 minutes

Cook Time: 30 minutes

Servings: 4 servings

Calories: 121kcal

Ingredients

• 8 oz white mushrooms slashed

• 1 onion, medium stripped and slashed

• 3 garlic cloves stripped and hacked

• 1 oz spread

• 2 tablespoon new tarragon hacked

• 2 cups vegetable or chicken stock

• 1 oz mascarpone cheddar

• 1 teaspoon salt

• 1 teaspoon dark pepper

Directions

1. In a pot heat the spread on a medium warmth

2. Cook the onion and the garlic for 5 min.

3. Add the mushrooms and tenderly Cook for 5 minutes. Spread with a cover to ensured the mushroom juices turn out.

4. Season with the salt and pepper.

5. Add the stock and mix well.

6. Add the new tarragon and stew for 15 minutes.

7. Stir in the mascarpone cheddar.

8. Either fill in as stout or fill a blender and mix for a smooth soup.

Notes

Mascarpone can be subbed with overwhelming cream or coconut cream.

The net carbs will be the Total carb check less the fibre tally. Carb check prohibits sugar alcohols.

Varieties may happen for different reasons, including item accessibility and food Preparation. We make no portrayal or guarantee of the precision of this data.

Nutrition

Serving: 1serving | Calories: 121kcal | Carbohydrates: 7.4g | Protein: 3.1g | Fat: 9.3g | Fiber: 1.9g

KETO CAFFLE BREAKFAST AND BRUNCH RECIPES

1. KETO COCONUT FLOUR WAFFLES RECIPE

This easy coconut flour waffles formula takes only 5 minutes to Prep + 5 minutes to Cook! Keto waffles with coconut flour make a delectable, without nut low carb breakfast.

Course Breakfast

Cooking American

Calories 474 kcal

Prep Time 5 minutes

Cook Time 5 minutes

Total Time 10 minutes

INGREDIENTS

♣ 3 tbsp Coconut flour

♣ 3 huge Eggs

♣ 2 oz Cream cheddar

♣ 2 tbsp of butter (or coconut oil)

♣ 1/4 cup of the Heavy cream (or any milk you like)

♣ 1 tbsp Erythritol (or any sugar)

♣ 1/2 tsp sans gluten heating powder

♣ 1/4 tsp Xanthan gum (discretionary, however, helps keep it together better)

♣ 1/2 tsp Vanilla concentrate (discretionary)

Directions

1. Preheat your waffle creator.

2. Combine all ingredients in a blender. Puree until smooth.

3. Let the hitter sit for a couple of moments to thicken. It ought to be thicker than a pourable hitter, however easy to spread. In the event that it's brittle like treat mixture, include more milk or cream, a tablespoon at once, until it's increasingly similar to a thick hitter.

4. Scoop a meagre 1 cup (128 grams) player into the waffle producer, spread and spread. Cook, as indicated by producer guidelines (for the most part around 4-5 minutes), or until steam, is never again turning out the sides. Cautiously expel the waffle from the iron (it's delicate while it's hot).

5. Repeat with the residual hitter.

6. Optional advance: For crisper waffles, heat them in the broiler on a stove safe cooling rack for two or three minutes at 400 degrees F (204 degrees C), or in a toaster broiler.
Formula NOTES

Serving size: 1 enormous Belgian waffle

NUTRITION INFORMATION PER SERVING

Nutrition Facts

Sum per serving. Serving size in formula notes above.

Calories474

Fat41g

Protein14g

Total Carbs10g

Net Carbs7g

Fiber3g

Sugar3g

2. MOMENT POT SOUS VIDE EGG BITES RECIPE

This 4-fixing, easy Instant Pot sous vide egg nibbles formula is much the same as Starbucks! Perceive how to make sous vide egg chomps in the Instant Pot, including bacon gruyere and different flavours.

Course Breakfast

Food French

Calories 227 kcal

Prep Time 10 minutes

Cook Time 9 minutes

Total Time 19 minutes

Servings egg nibbles

INGREDIENTS5 enormous Eggs

♣ 1/2 cup Gruyere cheddar (destroyed)

♣ 1/3 cup Heavy cream

♣ 2 tbsp Water (in addition to 1 cup more to fill the Instant Pot)

♣ 1/8 tsp Sea salt

♣ 1/8 tsp Black pepper

♣ 7 cuts Bacon (Cooked)

Guidelines

1. Grease a silicone egg nibble form with margarine or olive oil.

2. Stack the bacon cuts and cut them down the middle. Spot 2 bits of bacon next to each other into the base of the form, bending up the sides.

3. Blend the eggs, cheddar, cream, 2 tablespoons (29 ml) water, ocean salt, and dark pepper in a blender at rapid, until smooth and somewhat foamy. (Then again, you can utilize a hand blender in a bowl.)

4. Pour the egg blend equally into the moulds. Spread the shaping plate firmly with foil.

5. Pour 1 cup approximately (236 ml) of water into the Instant Pot and spot the trivet with handles inside. Cautiously place the egg chomp shape onto the trivet. Close the cover, set the steam valve to Seal, press the Manual catch, and set the time to 9 minutes at High weight.

6. When time is up, sit tight for 5 minutes of normal steam discharge.

7. Use broiler gloves to lift the trivet out of the weight Cooker. Evacuate the thwart and allow them to cool for 5 minutes (they will contract), at that point flip the form over a plate and jump out.

Formula NOTES

Serving size: 1 egg chomp

NUTRITION INFORMATION PER SERVING

Nutrition Facts

Sum per serving. Serving size in formula notes above.

Calories227

Fat20g

Protein11g

Total Carbs1g

Net Carbs0g

Fiber1g

Sugar1g

3. THE LOW CARB PALEO KETO BLUEBERRY AND THE MUFFINS RECIPE WITH ALMOND FLOUR

Perceive how to make the best keto biscuits in only 30 minutes! These ultra sodden almond flour blueberry biscuits without any Preparation are brisk and easy. It's the ideal low carb paleo blueberry biscuits formula - and the just a single you'll ever require.

Course Breakfast, Snack

Cooking American

Calories 217 kcal

Prep Time 10 minutes

Cook Time 20 minutes

Total Time 30 minutes

Servings biscuits

INGREDIENTS

♣ 2 1/2 cup Blanched almond flour

♣ 1/2 cup Erythritol (or any granulated sugar)

♣ 1 1/2 tsp without gluten heating powder

♣ 1/4 tsp Sea salt (discretionary, yet prescribed)

♣ 1/3 cup Coconut oil (estimated strong, at that point liquefied; can likewise utilize margarine)

♣ 1/3 cup Unsweetened almond milk

♣ 3 huge Eggs

♣ 1/2 tsp Vanilla concentrate

♣ 3/4 cup Blueberries

Directions

Snap-on the times in the directions below to begin a kitchen timer while you Cook.

1. Pre-heat the stove to 350 degrees F (177 degrees C). Line a biscuit skillet with 10 or 12 silicone or material paper biscuit liners. (Utilize 12 for lower calories/carbs, or 10 for bigger biscuit tops.)

2. In an enormous bowl, mix together the almond flour, erythritol, Preparing powder and ocean salt.

3. Mix in the softened coconut oil, almond milk, eggs, and vanilla concentrate—crease in the blueberries.

4. Distribute the hitter equally among the biscuit cups. Heat for around 20-25 minutes, until the top is brilliant and an embedded toothpick tells the truth.

Formula NOTES

Serving size: 1 biscuit

NUTRITION INFORMATION PER SERVING

Nutrition Facts

Sum per serving. Serving size in formula notes above.

Calories217

Fat19g

Protein7g

Total Carbs6g

Net Carbs3g

Fiber3g

Sugar2g

4. KETO MATCHA GREEN TEA FRAPPE RECIPE

Perceive how to make a matcha green tea frappe at home with only 5 ingredients + 5 minutes! My easy keto green tea frappe formula is without sugar, yet tastes simply like the bistro ones.

Course Breakfast, Drinks

Food American

Calories 156 kcal

Cook Time 5 minutes

Total Time 5 minutes

Servings serving

INGREDIENTS

♣ 3/4 cup of unsweetened almond milk (or coconut milk for sans nut)

♣ 2 tbsp of heavy cream

♣ 1/2 tbsp of Zulay Kitchen Matcha Green Tea

♣ 1 cup of Ice

♣ 1 tbsp Powdered erythritol (or any fluid or powdered sugar, discretionary)

♣ 1/2 tsp Vanilla concentrate (discretionary)

♣ Whipped cream (discretionary, for fixing - utilize natively constructed without sugar)

Directions

.

1. Combine everything with the exception of whipped cream in a blender. Mix until wanted consistency is come to.

2. If wanted, modify sugar or matcha to taste.

3. Pour into a glass or container. Top with whipped cream.

Formula NOTES

Serving size: 12 ounces (whole formula)

NUTRITION INFORMATION PER SERVING

Nutrition Facts

Sum per serving. Serving size in formula notes above.

Calories156

Fat13g

Protein5g

Total Carbs2g

Net Carbs2g

Fiber0g

Sugar1g

5. KETO PUMPKIN SPICE LATTE RECIPE

My mystery stunt for how to make a healthy pumpkin flavour latte at home, in only 5 minutes! This healthy KETO pumpkin zest latte formula suggests a flavour like one from a café, without the sugar. You'll never figure this is a low carb without sugar pumpkin flavour latte.

Course Breakfast, Snack

Food American

Calories 144 kcal

Prep Time 2 minutes

Cook Time 3 minutes

Total Time 5 minutes

Servings pumpkin zest latte

INGREDIENTS

♣ 3/4 cup of almond milk

♣ 2 tbsp of Heavy cream

♣ 2 tbsp pumpkin puree

♣ 2 tsp Xylitol (or other sugar of decision, to taste)

♣ 1/4 tsp Pumpkin pie zest (in addition to additional for sprinkling)

♣ 1/4 tsp Vanilla concentrate

♣ 1/2 cup Brewed solid espresso (or 1/4 mug coffee)

♣ Whipped cream (for serving)

Guidelines

1. Microwave technique: Stir together the almond milk, substantial cream, pumpkin puree, xylitol, and pumpkin pie zest in a 12-ounce mug. Microwave it for about 45 to 60 seconds, until hot.

Stove-top technique: Stir together the almond milk, substantial cream, pumpkin puree, xylitol, and pumpkin pie zest in a little pot, until hot. Fill a 12-ounce mug.

2. Add the vanilla concentrate. Utilize a milk frother to mix until the blend is smooth and foamy, and sugar has disintegrated.

3. Stir in the blended espresso. Top it up with the whipped cream and a sprinkle of pumpkin pie zest (discretionary).

Formula NOTES

Serving size: 1 pumpkin flavour latte

NUTRITION INFORMATION PER SERVING

Nutrition Facts

Sum per serving. Serving size in formula notes above.

Calories144

Fat13g

Protein2g

Total Carbs4g

Net Carbs3g

Fiber1g

Sugar2g

HEALTHY KETO ZUCCHINI PANCAKES RECIPE

Perceive how to make a healthy zucchini flapjacks formula in only 20 minutes, with 6 ingredients! Keto squash hotcakes are fleecy, flavorful, and delightful.

Course Breakfast, Main Course

Food Russian

Calories 204 kcal

Prep Time 10 minutes

Cook Time 10 minutes

Total Time 20 minutes

Servings

INGREDIENTS

♣ 3 cups Yellow squash or zucchini (ground)

♣ 1 tsp Sea salt (isolated)

♣ 3 enormous Egg

♣ 1/2 cup Full-fat buttermilk (or full-fat kefir)

♣ 3/4 cup Blanched almond flour

♣ 1/2 tsp Baking pop

♣ Olive oil (or any oil of decision for singing)

Directions

Snap-on the times in the directions below to begin a kitchen timer while you Cook.

1. Set the ground squash in a colander over the sink and sprinkle with 1/2 teaspoon ocean salt. Let it sit for in any event 10 minutes

2. Wrap the zucchini into a kitchen towel and bend over the sink to wring out any additional water. Attempt to discharge however much as could reasonably be expected, until the remaining ground zucchini is dry and not watery.

3. In a huge bowl, consolidate the almond flour, Preparing pop, and staying 1/2 teaspoon ocean salt. Beat in the eggs. Mix in buttermilk and squash.

4. Pour inadequate 1/4-cup-size (60 mL) circles of the hitter onto the container. Spread and Cook for 2-3 minutes, until the base is brilliant and edges are dry. Flip and rehash on the opposite side.

Formula NOTES

Serving size: 3 enormous flapjacks

NUTRITION INFORMATION PER SERVING

Nutrition Facts

Sum per serving. Serving size in formula notes above.

Calories204

Fat15g

Protein10g

Total Carbs8g

Net Carbs5g

Fiber3g

Sugar4g

7. LOW CARB CHOCOLATE PROTEIN PANCAKES RECIPE

Figure out how to make protein hotcakes! This low carb chocolate protein flapjacks formula (protein powder hotcakes) takes only 20 minutes and has 11g protein per serving.

Course Breakfast

Food American

Calories 237 kcal

Prep Time 10 minutes

Cook Time 10 minutes

Total Time 20 minutes

Servings

INGREDIENTS

♣ 1/2 cup of Whey protein powder (or collagen, or egg white protein powder)

♣ 1/2 cup of blanched almond flour

♣ 3 tbsp of cocoa powder

♣ 3 tbsp of erythritol (or sugar of decision)

♣ 1 tsp sans of gluten Preparing powder

♣ 4 big eggs

♣ 1/3 cup of almond milk

♣ 2 tbsp of Avocado oil (or liquefied coconut oil)

♣ 1 tsp of vanilla concentrate

♣ 1/8 tsp of sea salt

Guidelines

1. Shake all the ingredients together in the Whiskware Batter Mixer. Let the player sit for 5 minutes.

2. Preheat a dish over medium-low warmth. Crush player into the container to shape little circles (3 crawls in width). Spread with a top and Cook for two or three minutes, until bubbles structure on top. Utilize an exceptionally slim turner to deliberately flip the hotcakes, at that point Cook for two or three minutes on the opposite side.

3. Repeat with the rest of the player.

NUTRITION INFORMATION PER SERVING

Nutrition Facts

Sum per serving. Serving size in formula notes above.

Calories237

Fat20g

Protein11g

Total Carbs7g

Net Carbs5g

Fiber2g

Sugar0g

8. EASY VANILLA LOW CARB PROTEIN WAFFLES RECIPE

How to make protein waffles? EASY! This low carb high protein waffles formula (protein powder waffles) is only 5 ingredients and Prepared in under 10 minutes!

Course Breakfast

Food American

Calories 439 kcal

Prep Time 2 minutes

Cook Time 5 minutes

Total Time 7 minutes

Servings

INGREDIENTS

♣ 2 scoops Atkins Vanilla Protein Powder (1/4 cup)

♣ 2 tbsp Peanut margarine (smooth, no sugar included)

♣ 2 tbsp Coconut oil (softened)

♣ 3 enormous Eggs

♣ 1/2 tsp sans gluten Preparing powder

♣ 1/4 tsp Sea salt

Guidelines

1. Incoporate the ingredients into a blender, and mix until smooth.

2. Preheat your waffle iron. Move the player into the waffle iron (it will be thick) and appropriate equally.

3. Cook as indicated by producer's directions. Regularly the waffle Cooks for 4-5 minutes, and is done when steam is never again turning out.

Formula NOTES

Serving size: 1/2 enormous Belgian waffle

NUTRITION INFORMATION PER SERVING

Nutrition Facts

Sum per serving. Serving size in formula notes above.

Calories439

Fat32g

Protein29g

Total Carbs11g

Net Carbs5g

Fiber6g

Sugar2g

9. Immaculate BAKED HARD BOILED EGGS IN THE OVEN

Cooking eggs in the stove is EASY! Prepared hard bubbled eggs in the broiler take 20-30 minutes. For both delicate or hard bubbled eggs, here's a TIME CHART for how to bubble eggs in the stove.

Course Breakfast

Cooking American

Calories 70 kcal

Cook Time 30 minutes

Total Time 30 minutes

Servings 12 eggs

INGREDIENTS

♣ 12 huge Eggs

Directions

1. Preheat the stove to 325 degrees F (163 degrees C).

2. Place 1 egg in every cup in a biscuit tin.

3. Bake the eggs for 20 to 30 min. for your ideal degree of doneness. Eggs in the stove will take 20 minutes for delicate bubbled, 30 minutes for completely hard bubbled. See the diagram in the post above for Preparing times in the middle.

4. Meanwhile, Prepare a pot of ice water. When you expel the eggs from the broiler.

Formula NOTES

Serving size: 1 egg

NUTRITION INFORMATION PER SERVING

Nutrition Facts

Sum per serving. Serving size in formula notes above.

Calories70

Fat5g

Protein7g

Total Carbs0g

Net Carbs0g

Fiber0g

Sugar0g

10. EASY LOW CARB-KETO OATMEAL RECIPE

Figure out how to make keto oatmeal 4 different ways - maple walnut, strawberries and cream, chocolate nutty spread, or cinnamon roll - all dependent on an easy low carb oatmeal formula with 5 ingredients!

Course Breakfast

Cooking American

Calories 592 kcal

Prep Time 5 minutes

Cook Time 3 minutes

Total Time 8 minutes

Servings serving

INGREDIENTS

Basic Keto Oatmeal

- ♣ 1/4 cup Hemp seeds (hulled hemp seeds)

- ♣ 1 tbsp Golden flaxseed meal

- ♣ 1 tbsp Vital Proteins Collagen Peptides

- ♣ 1/2 tbsp Chia seeds

- ♣ 1/2 cup of coconut milk (from a bowl; 1/2 fluid and 1/2 thick cream; or simply overwhelming cream if not without dairy)

Discretionary Add-Ins (Recommended for all varieties)

- ♣ 1 tbsp Erythritol (to taste)

- ♣ 1 squeeze Sea salt (to taste)

Maple Pecan Add-Ins

♣ 1/2 tsp Maple extricate

♣ 2 tbsp Pecans (hacked)

Chocolate Peanut Butter Add-Ins

♣ 1 tbsp Peanut spread

♣ 1 tbsp Coconut milk (or almond milk)

♣ 1 tbsp without sugar dull chocolate chips

Strawberries and Cream Add-Ins

♣ 2 tbsp Strawberries (finely hacked)

♣ 1/2 tsp Vanilla concentrate

♣ 2 tbsp Coconut cream (or simply the cream part from canned coconut milk, or overwhelming cream if not without dairy)

Cinnamon Roll Add-Ins

♣ 3/4 tsp Cinnamon

♣ 3/4 tsp Vanilla concentrate (separated into 1/2 tsp and 1/4 tsp)

♣ 1 tbsp Powdered erythritol

♣ 1/2 tbsp Coconut cream (or simply the cream part from canned coconut milk, or overwhelming cream if not without dairy)

Directions

Basic Keto Oatmeal

1. Stir all ingredients, with the exception of cream or milk, together in a little pot. (This incorporates the discretionary sugar and salt if utilizing.)

2. Add cream/milk and speed until smooth.

3. Stovetop directions:

Stew for a couple of moments, until thickened.

Microwave guidelines:

Rather than a pan, utilize a microwave-safe bowl. Warmth for 1 to 2 minutes, until thickened.

Serve quickly, or follow choices below for include ins.

Maple Pecan Keto Oatmeal

1. Stir in the maple extricate and cleaved walnuts.

Chocolate Peanut Butter Keto Oatmeal

1. Stir in the nutty spread and additional milk, at that point stew for one more moment.

2. Stir in chocolate chips.

Strawberries and Cream Keto Oatmeal

1. Stir in strawberries, coconut cream, and vanilla concentrate.

Cinnamon Roll Keto Oatmeal

1. Stir in cinnamon and 1/2 tsp (2.5 mL) vanilla concentrate.

2. In an extremely little bowl, whisk together powdered sugar, coconut cream, and 1/4 tsp (1.25 mL) vanilla concentrate—shower over oatmeal in a twirling design.

Formula NOTES

Serving size: 1 formula

Nutrition information recorded does exclude the varieties - simply the basic formula.

NUTRITION INFORMATION PER SERVING

Nutrition Facts

Sum per serving. Serving size in formula notes above.

Calories592

Fat47g

Protein31g

Total Carbs9g

Net Carbs4g

Fiber5g

Sugar1g

11. LOW CARB DOUBLE CHOCOLATE PROTEIN MUFFINS RECIPE

These low carb twofold chocolate protein biscuits are easy to make, damp and heavenly. This healthy protein biscuit formula needs only 10 minutes Prep time!

Course Breakfast, Dessert

Cooking American

Calories 233 kcal

Prep Time 10 minutes

Cook Time 25 minutes

Total Time 35 minutes

Servings biscuits

INGREDIENTS

Snap underlined ingredients to get them!

♣ 2 cup Blanched almond flour

♣ 2/3 cup Allulose (or any granulated sugar)

♣ 1/2 cup Cocoa powder

♣ 1/4 cup Vital Proteins Collagen Peptides

♣ 1 1/2 tsp sans gluten heating powder

♣ 1/4 tsp Sea salt

♣ 1/3 cup Coconut oil

♣ 1/2 cup Unsweetened almond milk

♣ 3 enormous Eggs

♣ 1/2 tsp Vanilla concentrate

♣ 3/4 cup sans sugar dim chocolate chips

Guidelines

1. Preheat the broiler to 350 degrees F (177 degrees C). Line a biscuit container with 12 material paper liners or silicone biscuit liners.

2. In an enormous bowl, mix together the almond flour, sugar, cocoa powder, collagen peptides, Preparing powder and ocean salt.

3. Stir in the liquefied coconut oil and almond milk. Rush in the eggs and vanilla. Overlap in the chocolate chips last. (On the off chance that you'd like, you can save 1/4 cup of the chocolate chips to add on top.)

4. Scoop the player equally into the biscuit cups, filling practically full. On the off chance that you held some chocolate contributes the past advance, sprinkle them on top and press delicately into the player.

5. Bake it for 25 min., until the tops are brilliant and an embedded toothpick tells the truth.

Formula NOTES

Serving size: 1 biscuit

NUTRITION INFORMATION PER SERVING

Nutrition Facts

Sum per serving. Serving size in formula notes above.

Calories233

Fat20g

Protein10g

Total Carbs10g

Net Carbs5g

Fiber5g

Sugar0g

12. CHOCOLATE CHIP LOW CARB PALEO ZUCCHINI MUFFINS RECIPE

For the most delightful low carb zucchini biscuits or paleo zucchini biscuits, attempt this chocolate chip zucchini biscuits formula with coconut flour! It's sans sugar, keto, sans nut, and without dairy.

Course Breakfast, Dessert

Cooking American

Calories 181 kcal

Prep Time 10 minutes

Cook Time 35 minutes

Total Time 45 minutes
Servings biscuits

INGREDIENTS

Snap underlined ingredients to get them!

♣ 3/4 cup Coconut flour

♣ 1/2 cup Erythritol

♣ 2 tsp without gluten Preparing powder

♣ 1/4 tsp Sea salt

♣ 8 oz Zucchini (destroyed/ground, around 2 cups)

♣ 6 huge Egg

♣ 1/2 tsp Vanilla concentrate

♣ 2/3 cup Ghee (estimated strong, at that point liquefied; can likewise utilize without dairy spread enhanced coconut oil)

♣ 1/2 cup sans sugar dim chocolate chips

Guidelines

1. Preheat the broiler to 350 degrees F (177 degrees C). Line a biscuit skillet with 12 material paper liners.

2. In an enormous bowl, mix together the coconut flour, sugar, heating powder, and ocean salt.

3. Add the destroyed zucchini, eggs, and vanilla. Mix together until joined. Include the softened coconut oil and mix again until smooth.

4. Fold in the chocolate chips. Let the player sit for 5 minutes to thicken.

5. Divide the hitter among the material liners, filling them right to the top. Whenever wanted, you can spot the tops with more chocolate chips.

6. Bake for around 35 minutes, until brilliant and firm on top. Cool to room temperature in the dish, at that point on a wire rack. You can eat them warm, yet the surface is better in the event that you let them cool first.

Formula NOTES

Serving size: 1 biscuit

NUTRITION INFORMATION PER SERVING

Nutrition Facts

Sum per serving. Serving size in formula notes above.

Calories181

Fat15g

Protein5g

Total Carbs8g

Net Carbs4g

Fiber4g

Sugar1g

13. LOW CARB-CHOCOLATE CHIP PEANUT BUTTER PROTEIN COOKIES RECIPE

This easy chocolate chip nutty spread protein Cookies formula is so chewy. Only the 6 ingredients, 1 bowl, and 10 minutes Prep for delectable, flourless low carb protein Cookies. They're normally without gluten.

Course Breakfast, Dessert

Cooking American

Calories 118 kcal

Prep Time 10 minutes

Cook Time 20 minutes

Total Time 30 minutes

Servings Cookies

INGREDIENTS

♣ 1/3 cup Vital Proteins Collagen Peptides

♣ 1/2 cup Erythritol (or any granulated sugar)

♣ 1/4 tsp Sea salt

♣ 1 cup Peanut margarine (no sugar included)

♣ 2 enormous Eggs

♣ 1 tsp Vanilla concentrate

♣ 1/3 cup sans sugar dim chocolate chips

Guidelines

1. Preheat the broiler to 350 degrees F (177 degrees C). Line a heating sheet with material paper.

2. In a huge bowl, mix together the collagen, sugar, and ocean salt.

3. Add the egg and rush at the edge of the bowl to blend the yolk and white, before blending in with the dry ingredients. Include the nutty spread and vanilla, and mix until smooth.

4. Fold in the chocolate chips.

5. Scoop the treat batter utilizing a medium treat scoop, and press the mixture into it before discharging onto the lined Preparing sheet. Squash the treat mixture balls with the palm of your hand or the base of a wet glass, to around 1/4 in (~1/2 cm) thickness.

6. Bake this recipes for 16-20 min., until the Cookies are semi-firm and not clingy on top. Cool Totally to solidify more.

Formula NOTES

Serving size: 1 treat

NUTRITION INFORMATION PER SERVING

Nutrition Facts

Sum per serving. Serving size in formula notes above.

Calories118

Fat8g

Protein7g

Total Carbs4g

Net Carbs2g

Fiber2g

Sugar0g

14. HEALTHY CHOCOLATE PEANUT BUTTER LOW CARB SMOOTHIE RECIPE

This keto chocolate nutty spread smoothie formula will be one of your fave healthy low carb smoothies. So rich, and Prepared in a short time with 5 ingredients!

Course Breakfast, Drinks

Cooking American

Calories 435 kcal

Prep Time 5 minutes

Total Time 5 minutes

Servings (1 cup each)

INGREDIENTS

Snap underlined ingredients to get them!

- ♣ 1/4 cup Peanut spread (rich)

- ♣ 3 tbsp Cocoa powder

- ♣ 1 cup of heavy cream (or coconut cream for without dairy or veggie lover)

- ♣ 1 1/2 cup unsweetened almond milk (ordinary or vanilla)

- ♣ 6 tbsp Powdered erythritol (to taste)

- ♣ 1/8 tsp Sea salt (discretionary)

Directions

1. Combine all ingredients in a blender.

2. Puree until smooth. Modify sugar to taste whenever wanted.

Formula NOTES

Serving size: 1 cup

NUTRITION INFORMATION PER SERVING

Nutrition Facts

Sum per serving. Serving size in formula notes above.

Calories435

Fat41g

Protein9g

Total Carbs10g

Net Carbs6g

Fiber4g

Sugar3g

15. FATHEAD KETO CINNAMON ROLLS RECIPE - QUICK and EASY

Everybody cherishes these keto cinnamon rolls! Just 40 minutes to make, with basic ingredients (no exceptional flour!), and they're Totally tasty. For a stunning low carb dessert or keto breakfast, attempt this fathead cinnamon moves formula.

Course Breakfast, Dessert

Food American

Calories 321 kcal

Prep Time 20 minutes

Cook Time 20 minutes

Total Time 40 minutes

Servings cinnamon rolls

INGREDIENTS

♣ 2 cup Macadamia nuts (10 oz)

♣ 1/4 cup Erythritol

♣ 1 tbsp sans gluten heating powder

♣ 2 enormous Egg

♣ 1 tsp Vanilla concentrate (discretionary)

♣ 4 cup Mozzarella cheddar (destroyed)

♣ 4 oz Cream cheddar

Filling

♣ 1/4 cup Butter (softened)

♣ 1/2 cup Erythritol

♣ 2 tbsp Cinnamon

Icing

♣ 1/3 cup sans sugar cream cheddar icing

♣ 1 tbsp of almond milk (or any milk of decision)

Directions

1. Put the macadamia nuts into a food processor fitted with a S blade sharp edge. Heartbeat just until the nuts arrive at a fine, brittle consistency, without huge pieces. Make a point to beat, don't leave the food processor running, to attempt to make flour and not nut margarine. Scratch the sides varying. The nuts may, in any case, start to shape nut margarine a bit, however, attempt to stay away from however much as could be expected.

2. Add the erythritol and heating powder. Heartbeat a few times, just until blended.

3. Add the eggs and vanilla. Heartbeat several times once more, just until blended.

4. Heat the mozzarella and cream cheddar in the microwave for around 2 minutes, blending part of the way through and toward the end, or on the stove in a twofold evaporator, until easy to mix. Mix until smooth.

5. Add the cheddar blend to the food processor. Push the cheddar blend down into the nut/egg blend. Heartbeat/puree until uniform mixture structures, scratching down the sides vary. If you experience difficulty getting it to blend, you can massage a little with a spatula and afterwards beat some more.

6. Refrigerate the batter directly in the food processor for around 30-an hour, until the top is firm and not clingy.

7. Meanwhile, preheat the stove to 375 degrees F (191 degrees C). Line a 9x13 in (23x33 cm) heating container with material paper.

8. Take the batter out onto an enormous bit of material paper (not the one on the heating sheet). It will, in any case, be genuinely clingy. Utilize a tad of the softened margarine on your hands to forestall staying as you spread it into a square shape.

9. Brush the mixture square shape with the majority of the staying softened margarine, leaving aside around 1-2 tablespoons. Mix together the erythritol and cinnamon for the filling. Sprinkle the blend uniformly over the square shape.

10. Oil your hands again with the softened spread. Beginning from a long side of the square shape, fold up the mixture into a log. As you come, oil the underside of the log as you strip it away from the material underneath during rolling. (This is to forestall breaking and staying.)

11. Slice the sign into 1 in (2.5 cm) thick cuts, which will look like pinwheels. Spot the pinwheels level onto the lined Preparing dish, practically contacting however not exactly.

12. Bake for around 25 minutes, until the keto cinnamon rolls are brilliant on top. Cool for in any event 20 minutes, until firm.
13. Meanwhile, making the icing. Beat almond milk into the icing a tablespoon at once, until the icing is sufficiently slender to shower. When the keto cinnamon rolls are sufficiently firm, sprinkle the icing over them.

Formula NOTES

Serving size: 1 cinnamon roll

NUTRITION INFORMATION PER SERVING

Nutrition Facts

Sum per serving. Serving size in formula notes above.

Calories321

Fat29.5g

Protein11g

Total Carbs5g

Net Carbs3g

Fiber2g

Sugar1g

16. EASY KETO ALMOND FLOUR PANCAKES RECIPE

These soft almond flour hotcakes are so easy to make! Only a couple of basic ingredients required. You're going to cherish this easy keto almond flour hotcake formula. They're paleo, as well!

Course Breakfast, Main Course

Cooking American

Calories 261 kcal

Prep Time 5 minutes

Cook Time 15 minutes

Total Time 20 minutes

Servings

This video can't be played on account of a specialized error. (Error Code: 100000)

INGREDIENTS

♣ 1 cup Blanched almond flour

♣ 2 tbsp Erythritol (or any sugar; use coconut sugar for paleo)

♣ 1 tsp sans gluten heating powder

♣ 1/8 tsp Sea salt

♣ 2 eggs

♣ 1/3 cup of unsweetened almond milk (or any milk of decision)

♣ 2 tbsp Avocado oil (or any nonpartisan oil of decision; in addition to additional for singing)

♣ 1 tsp Vanilla concentrate (discretionary)

Directions

1. Mix the ingredients together in a can until smooth.

2. Preheat an oiled dish on the stove at medium-low warmth. Pour circles of player onto the dish, 1/8 cup (30 mL) at once for 3 in (8 cm) flapjacks. Spread and Cook around 1/2 to 2 minutes, until bubbles begin to frame on the edges. Flip and Cook one more moment or two, until seared on the opposite side.

3. Repeat with the rest of the hitter.

Formula NOTES

Serving size: 3-inch flapjacks

NUTRITION INFORMATION PER SERVING

Nutrition Facts

Sum per serving. Serving size in formula notes above.

Calories261

Fat23g

Protein9g

Total Carbs6g

Net Carbs4g

Fiber2g

Sugar1g

AT LEAST 15 RECIPES FOR LUNCH AND DINNER (IMPORTANT: BURGERS, HOT DOG, PIZZA)

1.   LOW CARB KETO CABBAGE ROLLS RECIPE WITHOUT RICE

Perceive how to make cabbage moves without rice that are similarly as delightful! This easy, whole30, low carb keto cabbage moves formula is comfort food reconsidered.

Course Main Course

Food Polish

Calories 321 kcal

Prep Time 25 minutes

Cook Time 60 minutes

Total Time 1 hour 25 minutes

Servings

INGREDIENTS

☐   1 head Cabbage

- ☐ 1 lb ground hamburger

- ☐ 1 14.5-oz can Diced tomatoes (depleted)

- ☐ 1 enormous Egg

- ☐ 4 cloves Garlic (minced)

- ☐ 2 tsp Italian flavouring

- ☐ 1 tsp Sea salt

- ☐ 1/4 tsp Black pepper

- ☐ 1 cup Cauliflower rice

- ☐ 1 15-oz would tomato be able to sauce

Guidelines

1.   Preheat the broiler to 350 degrees F (177 degrees C).

2.   Bring an enormous pot of water to a bubble. Include the head of cabbage into the bubbling water, drenching completely. Bubble for 5-8 minutes, just until the leaves are sufficiently delicate to twist. They will turn brilliant green, and the external leaves may fall off, which is alright and you can angle them out.

3.   Remove the cabbage from the bubbling water. Put aside to cool. Leave the boiling water in the pot until further notice, and you may require it again later when stripping the cabbage leaves.

4. Meanwhile, pan sears the cauliflower rice for a couple of moments as per the guidelines here.

5. In an enormous bowl, join the ground hamburger, diced tomatoes, egg, minced garlic, Italian flavouring, ocean salt, and dark pepper. Blend until simply consolidated, yet don't over-blend—overlap in the Cooked cauliflower rice. Put in a safe spot.

6. Spread the large part of the tomato sauce in an enormous rectangular or oval clay heating dish. Put in a safe spot.

7. Carefully strip the leaves from the cabbage. To do this, flip cabbage over such a centre side is up, and cut the leaves individually from the centre, at that point cautiously strip (they are delicate). Rather than stripping leaves back, slide your fingers between the layers of cabbage to discharge them. The leaves outwardly will be delicate and simpler to strip, yet inside they might be firmer. In the event that they are excessively firm and fresh to twist, you can restore the incompletely stripped cabbage to bubbling water for a couple more minutes to mollify more.

8. Cut the thick rib from the focal point of each cabbage leaf, cutting in a "V" shape. Spot 1/3 cup (67 grams) hamburger blend into a log shape toward one side of a cabbage leaf. Overlay in the sides, at that point, move up, similar to a burrito. Spot the cabbage move, crease side down, into the heating dish over the sauce. Rehash to make 12 cabbage rolls. (In the event that the inward leaves are excessively little, you may need to utilize two to cover them to fit the filling.)

9. Spread the Preparing dish firmly with foil. Bake for 60 minutes, or until the meat is Cooked through.

Formula NOTES

Serving size: 2 cabbage rolls

NUTRITION INFORMATION PER SERVING

Nutrition Facts

Sum per serving. We are serving size in formula notes above.

Calories321

Fat18g

Protein25g

Total Carbs15g

Net Carbs10g

Fiber5g

Sugar7g

2. KETO BUFFALO CHICKEN SPAGHETTI SQUASH CASSEROLE RECIPE

You need only 6 straightforward ingredients for keto bison chicken spaghetti squash goulash. Make this gooey spaghetti squash meal formula for a healthy, encouraging meal today around evening time!

Course Main Course

Food Dinner

Calories 301 kcal

Prep Time 15 minutes

Cook Time 40 minutes

Total Time 55 minutes

Servings

INGREDIENTS

- 1 medium Spaghetti squash

- 1 cup Blue cheddar dressing (in addition to additional for garnish)

- 1/4 cup Buffalo sauce (will be mellow; can add more to taste)

- 4 oz Cream cheddar (mellowed)

- 2 cups Shredded chicken (Cooked)

- 1 cup cheddar (destroyed)

- Green onions (discretionary, for garnish)

Guidelines

1.   Preheat the broiler to 400 degrees F (204 degrees C).

2.   Use a blade to jab a couple of openings everywhere throughout the spaghetti squash. Spot onto a heating sheet and Prepare for 30-40 minutes, until a blade goes in with almost no opposition. Expel from the stove (leave it on) and put in a safe spot.

3.   Meanwhile, in an enormous bowl, mix together the blue cheddar dressing, wild ox sauce, and cream cheddar. Mix in the destroyed chicken.

4.   Cut the spaghetti squash into equal parts and utilize a spoon to scoop out the seeds. Utilize a fork to discharge the strands into the bowl with the chicken blend. Mix together.

5.   Transfer the goulash blend to an enormous meal dish (12x8" oval dish, 2.4 qt.). Top with destroyed cheddar. Spot in the broiler for 10 minutes, until the cheddar dissolves.

6.   If wanted, shower the top with extra blue cheddar dressing and sprinkle with green onions.

Formula NOTES

Serving size: 1/3 cup or 1/6 of formula

NUTRITION INFORMATION PER SERVING

Nutrition Facts

Sum per serving. Serving size in formula notes above.

Calories301

Fat20g

Protein19g

Total Carbs14g

Net Carbs12g

Fiber2g

Sugar6g

3. CHIPOTLE BEEF BARBACOA RECIPE (SLOW COOKER/CROCKPOT)

The best Crock Pot barbacoa ever! On the off chance that you love barbacoa meat, you need to attempt this copycat Chipotle barbacoa formula in a slow Cooker. It's healthy, easy, low carb, and self-destruct tastily.

Course Main Course

Food American

Calories 242 kcal

Prep Time 10 minutes

Cook Time 4 hours

Total Time 4 hours 10 minutes

Serving

INGREDIENTS

☐ 3 lb Beef brisket or throw broil (cut and cut into 2-inch lumps)

☐ 1/2 cup Beef soup (or chicken stock)

☐ 2 medium Chipotle chiles in adobo (counting the sauce, around 4 tsp)

☐ 5 cloves Garlic (minced)

☐ 2 tbsp Apple juice vinegar

☐ 2 tbsp Lime juice

☐ 1 tbsp dried oregano

☐ 2 tsp Cumin

☐ 2 tsp Sea salt

☐ 1 tsp Black pepper

☐ 1/2 tsp Ground cloves (discretionary)

☐ 2 entire Bay leaf

Directions

Snap-on the times in the directions below to begin a kitchen timer while you Cook.

1.   Combine the soup, chipotle chiles in adobo sauce, garlic, apple juice vinegar, lime juice, dried oregano, cumin, ocean salt, dark pepper, and ground cloves in a blender (everything with the exception of the hamburger and cove leaves). Puree until smooth.

2.   Place the hamburger lumps in the slow Cooker. Pour the pureed blend from the blender on top. Include the (entire) cove leaves.

3.   Cook for 4-6 hrs. on high temp. or 8-10 hrs. on low, until the meat is self-destructed delicate.

4.   Remove the straight leaves. Shred the meat utilizing two forks and mix into the juices. Spread and rest for 5-10 minutes to allow the meat to ingest much more flavour. Utilize an opened spoon to serve.

Formula NOTES

Serving size: 1/3 lb, or 1/9 whole formula

NUTRITION INFORMATION PER SERVING

Nutrition Facts

Sum per serving. Serving size in formula notes above.

Calories242

Fat11g

Protein32g

Total Carbs2g

Net Carbs1g

Fiber1g

Sugar0.3g

Firm BAKED CHICKEN LEGS DRUMSTICKS RECIPE

This 10-minute-Prep easy stove broiled chicken drumsticks formula will make SUPER firm Prepared chicken legs that turn out splendidly inevitably! It's the main guide for how to Prepare chicken legs you'll ever require.

Course Main Course

Food American

Calories 236 kcal

Prep Time 10 minutes

Cook Time 40 minutes

Total Time 50 minutes

Servings

INGREDIENTS

- ☐   6 medium chicken drumsticks (~1 1/2 lb)

- ☐   1/4 cup butter (softened)

- ☐   1/2 tsp smoked paprika

- ☐   1/2 tsp Garlic powder

- ☐   1/2 tsp Sea salt

- ☐   1/4 tsp Black pepper

Guidelines

1.   Preheat the broiler to 425 degrees F (218 degrees C). Line a heating sheet with foil and spot a broiler-safe rack on top.

2.   Organize the chicken legs on the rack.

3.   Brush the chicken drumsticks with dissolved margarine—season with smoked paprika, garlic powder, salt and pepper.

4.   Bake the chicken legs in the stove for 25 minutes. Flip and heat for another 10-20 minutes, until the inner temperature comes to in any event 165 degrees F (74 degrees C).

Perusers ALSO MADE THESE KETO LOW CARB RECIPES

Formula NOTES

Serving size: 1 drumstick

NUTRITION INFORMATION PER SERVING

Nutrition Facts

Sum per serving. Serving size in formula notes above.

Calories236

Fat16g

Protein22g

Total Carbs0g

Net Carbs0g

Fiber0g

Sugar0g

5. ITALIAN STUFFED ARTICHOKES RECIPE WITH SAUSAGE

Figure out how to make stuffed artichokes in the broiler with bit by bit pictures! This Prepared Italian stuffed artichokes formula makes a tasty low carb meal or hors d'oeuvre.

Course Main Course

Cooking Italian

Calories 604 kcal

Prep Time 20 minutes

Cook Time 55 minutes

Total Time 1 hour 15 minutes

Servings

INGREDIENTS

Artichokes:

- ☐ 4 huge Ocean Mist Farms Artichokes

- ☐ 2 tbsp Lemon juice

- ☐ 2 tbsp Olive oil

- ☐ 2 tbsp Grated Parmesan cheddar (separated)

Filling:

- ☐ 1 lb Ground Italian Sausage

- ☐ 4 cloves Garlic (minced)

- ☐ 2 tsp Italian flavouring

- ☐ 1/2 cup Grated Parmesan cheddar (separated)

Directions

1.   Cut about an inch off the highest points of the artichokes and remove the stems to make a level base. Use kitchen shears to trim the sharp warns the leaves.

2.   Bring a huge pot of saltwater to a bubble. Include the artichokes and spot a warmth safe dish on them to keep them submerged in the water—bubble for 15 minutes. Evacuate and put aside topsy turvy to deplete and cool.

3.   Meanwhile, preheat the broiler to 375 degrees F (190 degrees C).

4.   In an enormous bowl, combine the Italian hotdog, minced garlic, Italian flavouring and 1/2 cup (50 grams) ground parmesan, until simply joined. Don't over-blend.

5.   Once the artichokes are sufficiently cool to deal with, dry them with paper towels, tenderly pry open the middle leaves, and utilize a spoon with a curving movement to scoop out the fluffy gag inside. Spot the artichokes into a stoneware heating dish, looking up.

6.   Drizzle the artichokes done with lemon juice and olive oil, including the tops and sides.

7.   Stuff every artichoke with the frankfurter blend, ensuring you get some between all the leaves and in the middle. Sprinkle the artichokes with the staying 2 tablespoons (30 grams) ground parmesan.

8.   Cover the heating dish with foil. Prepare for 40-50 minutes, until the hotdog is Cooked through (to an interior temperature of 165 degrees F (74 degrees C)) and the external leaves are easy to expel.

9.   Remove the foil. Set the stove to sear and put the stuffed artichokes under the oven for two or three minutes to dark-coloured the cheddar.

Perusers ALSO MADE THESE KETO LOW CARB RECIPES

Formula NOTES

Serving size: 1 stuffed artichoke*

*Nutrition data is expected for a full, filling meal. On the off chance that you are viewing carbs or calories, a large portion of a stuffed artichoke would, in any case, be a bounty for a serving. Serving size could be 1/8 or 1/4 of the stuffed artichoke as an hors d'oeuvre.

NUTRITION INFORMATION PER SERVING

Nutrition Facts

Sum per serving. Serving size in formula notes above.

Calories604

Fat47g

Protein28g

Total Carbs21g

Net Carbs12g

Fiber9g

Sugar2g

6. LOW CARB KETO CHEESY TACO SKILLET RECIPE

A keto mushy taco skillet formula in only 25 minutes, with 7 basic ingredients! This easy hamburger taco skillet dinner is ideal for occupied weeknights.

Course Main Course

Food Mexican

Calories 547 kcal

Cook Time 25 minutes

Total Time 25 minutes

Servings

Formula VIDEO

INGREDIENTS

- ☐ 1 lb ground hamburger

- ☐ 2 tbsp Taco flavouring

- ☐ 1/2 cup Water

- ☐ 1/2 enormous Onion (diced)

- ☐ 3 enormous Bell peppers (cut into 1-inch strips)

- ☐ 1 14.5-oz can Dice tomatoes (depleted well)

- ☐ 1 cup Mexican cheddar mix (destroyed)

☐   1/4 cup Green onions (cut)

Guidelines

1.   Heat a skillet over medium-high warmth. Include ground hamburger and Cook around 10 minutes, breaking separated the meat with a spatula or spoon, until seared.

2.   Add the taco flavouring and water. Cook for 2-3 minutes, until the additional water, is ingested or vanishes.

3.   Reduce warmth to medium. Include the onions and ringer peppers. Cook for 5-10 minutes, until onions are delicate and translucent.

4.   Add the diced tomatoes. Stew for a couple of moments, until hot and any additional dampness vanishes.

5.   Reduce warmth to low. Sprinkle destroyed cheddar on top. Spread with a cover and warmth just until the cheddar dissolves. Expel from warmth and top with green onions.

Perusers ALSO MADE THESE KETO LOW CARB RECIPES

Formula NOTES

Serving size: 1/2 cups, or 1/4 whole skillet*

*This is a liberal serving size. Contingent upon your requirements, you could separate the skillet into 6 servings rather than 4 for littler segments and 9g net carbs per serving.

NUTRITION INFORMATION PER SERVING

Nutrition Facts

Sum per serving. Serving size in formula notes above.

Calories547

Fat35g

Protein41g

Total Carbs17g

Net Carbs12g

Fiber5g

Sugar9g

7. SMOTHERED PORK CHOPS RECIPE WITH ONION GRAVY

A tasty, easy heated covered pork cleaves formula with onion sauce! Perceive how to make the juiciest covered pork slashes in the broiler, with only 7 ingredients.

Course Main Course

Food American

Calories 541 kcal

Prep Time 10 minutes

Cook Time 50 minutes

Total Time 60 minutes

Servings

INGREDIENTS

- ☐ 4 8-oz Boneless pork cleaves

- ☐ 1 tsp Sea salt

- ☐ 1/4 tsp Black pepper

- ☐ 2 tbsp Olive oil

- ☐ 1 enormous Onion (cut into slender half moons)

- ☐ 2 cloves of Garlic (minced)

- ☐

- ☐ 1 cup of Chicken juices

☐   1.5 oz of Cream cheddar (cut into little lumps)

Guidelines

1.   Season the pork slashes on the two sides with ocean salt, garlic powder, onion powder, and pepper.

2.   Heat the olive oil in a dutch broiler over medium-high warmth. Include the pork hacks and burn on the two sides, around 3 minutes for each side without moving, until seared. Move the pork slashes to a plate and put in a safe spot.

3.   Reduce warmth to medium-low or medium. Utilizing a similar dutch broiler, saute the cut onions for 15-20 minutes, until caramelized.

4.   Once the onions are caramelized, preheat the stove to 375 degrees F (190 degrees C).

5.   Saute for about a moment, until fragrant.

6.   Add the chicken soup to the dutch broiler—Scratch any caramelized bits from the base of the skillet. Bring to a delicate bubble, at that point stew for around 2-3 minutes, until it gets thicker and the volume is decreased by at any rate 1/4.

7.   Remove from heat. Include the cream cheddar. Mix in the cream cheddar until it dissolves into the sauce.

8.   Return the pork hacks to the dutch broiler and spoon the sauce and onions over them. Spread with the cover and Prepare for 20-25 minutes, until Cooked through.

Perusers ALSO MADE THESE KETO LOW CARB RECIPES

Formula NOTES

Serving size: 1 pork slash with gravy*

*Nutrition data is for huge, 8-ounce pork slashes. Contingent upon what you're serving them with, it might bode well to slice the serving size down the middle to 4 ounces.

NUTRITION INFORMATION PER SERVING

Nutrition Facts

Sum per serving. Serving size in formula notes above.

Calories541

Fat35g

Protein48g

Total Carbs5g

Net Carbs4g

Fiber1g

Sugar2g

8. LOW CARB KETO TURKEY MEATLOAF RECIPE

The entire family will adore this keto turkey meatloaf formula! Low carb bacon-wrapped turkey meatloaf is delightful, delicious, and takes only 10 minutes to Prep.

Course Main Course

Food American

Calories 241 kcal

Prep Time 10 minutes

Cook Time 50 minutes

Total Time 60 minutes

Servings

INGREDIENTS

Turkey Meatloaf:

☐   2 lb ground turkey

☐   1/2 enormous Onion (cleaved finely)

- [ ] 6 cloves Garlic (minced)

- [ ] 1/3 cup Tomato sauce

- [ ] 2 tsp Italian flavouring

- [ ] 1 1/2 tsp Sea salt

- [ ] 1/4 tsp Black pepper

- [ ] 1/2 cup Blanched almond flour

- [ ] 2 enormous Eggs

Beating:

- [ ] 10 cuts Bacon

- [ ] 1/4 cup sans sugar BBQ sauce

Guidelines.

1.   Preheat the broiler to 350 degrees F (177 degrees C). Line a Preparing sheet with foil or material paper.

2.   In an enormous bowl, consolidate all turkey meatloaf ingredients. Blend until simply consolidated - don't over blend.

3.   Form the ground turkey blend into a 10x6 inch portion on the lined heating sheet.

4.   Arrange the bacon cuts in a solitary layer on the meatloaf, going over the short way, and fold the closures underneath the sides of the meatloaf.

5.   Bake for 30 minutes.

6.   Spread the BBQ sauce and sides of the turkey meatloaf. Come back to the broiler and heat for 20-35 additional minutes, until Cooked through and inner temperature arrives at 160 degrees F (71 degrees C). (Time will shift contingent upon the thickness of the portion.) If wanted, place under the grill for a couple of moments to fresh up the bacon.

7.   Rest for 10 minutes before cutting utilizing a serrated blade.

Perusers ALSO MADE THESE KETO LOW CARB RECIPES

Formula NOTES

Serving size: 1 3/4-inch cut, or 1/12 whole meatloaf

NUTRITION INFORMATION PER SERVING

Nutrition Facts

Sum per serving. Serving size in formula notes above.

Calories241

Fat17g

Protein19g

Total Carbs4g

Net Carbs3g

Fiber1g

Sugar 1g

9.LOW CARB KETO CABBAGE ROLLS RECIPE WITHOUT RICE

Perceive how to make cabbage moves without rice that are similarly as flavorful! This easy, whole30, low carb keto cabbage moves formula is comfort food reconsidered.

Course Main Course

Cooking Polish

Calories 321 kcal

Prep Time 25 minutes

Cook Time 60 minutes

Total Time 1 hour 25 minutes

Servings

INGREDIENTS

- [ ] 1 head Cabbage

- [ ] 1 lb ground hamburger

- [ ] 1 14.5-oz can Diced tomatoes (depleted)

- [ ] 1 enormous Egg

- [ ] 4 cloves Garlic (minced)

- [ ] 2 tsp Italian flavouring

- [ ] 1 tsp Sea salt

- [ ] 1/4 tsp Black pepper

- [ ] 1 cup Cauliflower rice

- [ ] 1 15-oz would tomato be able to sauce

Guidelines

1.   Preheat the broiler to 350 degrees F (177 degrees C).

2.   Bring an enormous pot of water to a bubble. Include the head of cabbage into the bubbling water, inundating completely. Bubble for 5-8 minutes, just until the leaves are sufficiently delicate to twist. They will turn brilliant green, and the external leaves may fall off, which is alright and you can angle them out.

3.   Remove the cabbage from the bubbling water. Put aside to cool. Leave the heated water in the pot until further notice, and you may require it again later when stripping the cabbage leaves.

4.   Meanwhile, pan sears the cauliflower rice for a couple of moments as per the guidelines here.

5.   In an enormous bowl, join the ground hamburger, diced tomatoes, egg, minced garlic, Italian flavouring, ocean salt, and dark pepper. Blend until simply joined, yet don't over-blend—crease in the Cooked cauliflower rice. Put in a safe spot.

6.   Spread part of the tomato sauce in an enormous rectangular or oval artistic heating dish. Put in a safe spot.

7.   Carefully strip the leaves from the cabbage. To do this, flip cabbage over such a centre side is up, and cut the leaves individually from the centre, at that point cautiously strip (they are delicate). Rather than stripping leaves back, slide your fingers between the layers of cabbage to discharge them. The leaves outwardly will be delicate and simpler to strip, however inside they might be firmer. In the event that they are excessively firm and fresh to twist, you can restore the somewhat stripped cabbage to bubbling water for a couple more minutes to mollify more.

8.   Cut the thick rib from the focal point of each cabbage leaf, cutting in a "V" shape. Spot 1/3 cup (67 grams) meat blend into a log shape toward one side of a cabbage leaf. Overlay in the sides, at that point, move up, similar to a burrito. Spot the cabbage move, crease side down, into the Preparing dish over the sauce. Rehash to make 12 cabbage rolls. (In the event that the inward leaves are excessively little, you may need to utilize two to cover them to fit the filling.)

9.   Spread the Preparing dish firmly with foil—Bake for 60 minutes, or until the hamburger is Cooked through.

Perusers ALSO MADE THESE KETO LOW CARB RECIPES

Formula NOTES

Serving size: 2 cabbage rolls

Video Showing How To Make Cabbage Rolls:

Try not to miss the VIDEO above - it's the most effortless approach to figure out how to make Cabbage Rolls!

NUTRITION INFORMATION PER SERVING

Nutrition Facts

Sum per serving. Serving size in formula notes above.

Calories321

Fat18g

Protein25g

Total Carbs15g

Net Carbs10g

Fiber5g

Sugar7g

10.   KETO MEXICAN CHEESE and CHICKEN STUFFED POBLANO PEPPERS RECIPE

Perceive how to make Mexican keto stuffed poblano peppers with basic ingredients, in only 30 minutes! This mushy chicken stuffed poblano peppers formula is loaded with taco flavours.

Course dinner

Cooking Mexican

Calories 216 kcal

Prep Time 5 minutes

Cook Time 20 minutes

Total Time 25 minutes

Servings

INGREDIENTS

- [ ] 3 huge Poblano peppers

- [ ] 1 tbsp Butter

- [ ] 2 cloves Garlic (minced)

- [ ] 2 cups shredded chicken

- [ ] 1 14.5-oz can Diced tomatoes (NOT depleted)

- [ ] 2 tbsp Taco flavouring

- [ ] 3 oz Cream cheddar (cubed)

- [ ] 3/4 cup cheddar (destroyed)

- [ ] Cilantro (discretionary, for fixing)

Directions

.

1. Pre-heat the stove to 350 degrees F (177 degrees C).

2.   Cut the peppers down the middle and evacuate the seeds. Spot them onto a lined Preparing sheet. Put in a safe spot.

3.   In a skillet over medium warmth, liquefy the margarine. Include the garlic and saute for around 30 seconds, until fragrant.

4.   Add the destroyed chicken, diced tomatoes (with fluid), and taco flavouring. Heat the stew for 3-5 minutes, until the additional fluid is ingested into the chicken.

5.   Reduce warmth to low. Mix in the cream cheddar, squeezing with the rear of a spoon or spatula to assist it with blending in, until softened and smooth.

6.   Stuff it into the poblano peppers and spot, open side up, back onto the heating sheet. Sprinkle destroyed cheddar on each pepper half, around 2 tablespoons (28 grams) each.

7.   Bake for 15-20 minutes, until peppers are delicate and cheddar is softened. Embellishment with crisp cilantro whenever wanted.

Perusers ALSO MADE THESE KETO LOW CARB RECIPES

Formula NOTES

Serving size: 1 stuffed pepper

NUTRITION INFORMATION PER SERVING

Nutrition Facts

Sum per serving. Serving size in formula notes above.

Calories216

Fat15g

Protein16g

Total Carbs6g

Net Carbs4g

Fiber2g

Sugar3g

11. HALIBUT RECIPE WITH LEMON BUTTER SAUCE

This dish singed halibut formula with lemon margarine sauce takes only 20 minutes... which you'd never surmise with how extravagant seared halibut looks. I'll tell you the best way to container burn halibut, in addition to how to make the ideal sauce for halibut.

Course dinner, Main Course

Cooking American

Calories 513 kcal

Prep Time 5 minutes

Cook Time 10 minutes

Total Time 15 minutes

Servings

INGREDIENTS

- [ ] 4 6-oz of Halibut fillets (1.5 lb Total)

- [ ] 1/2 tsp of Garlic powder

- [ ] 1/2 tsp of Paprika

- [ ] 1 tsp of Sea salt

- [ ] 1/4 tsp of Black pepper

- [ ] 2 tbsp of Olive oil

Lemon spread sauce:

- [ ] 1/2 cup Salted spread

- [ ] 1 medium Lemon (cut down the middle)

Directions

1. Use paper towels to pat the halibut filets Totally dry - this will guarantee in any event, sautéing. Season the fish on the two sides with garlic powder, paprika, ocean salt, and dark pepper. Put in a safe spot.

2. Heat the olive oil in an enormous skillet over medium-high warmth for 2 minutes.

3. Add the fish filets in a solitary layer (you can do it in clumps if all the fish won't fit in a solitary layer). Burn, without moving, for 3-4 minutes, until the edges of the fish are misty.

4. Remove the fish from the container and spread firmly with foil to keep warm.

5. Reduce warmth to medium-low. Add the spread to a similar dish. Hang tight for it to dissolve, at that point heat for 2-3 minutes, mixing every so often, until the margarine is Cooked and smells nutty.

6. Use the Zulay Kitchen Lemon Squeezer to crush all the juice from the two parts of the lemon into the container. Bring to a stew, at that point diminish warmth and stew for around 3-4 minutes, frequently mixing, until the volume is decreased considerably. The lemon margarine sauce will, in any case, be slender.

7. Drizzle a little lemon margarine sauce over each serving plate. Spot the skillet burned halibut filets over the sauce, at that point shower more sauce on top.

Perusers ALSO MADE THESE KETO LOW CARB RECIPES

Formula NOTES

Serving size: 1 halibut filet + 2 tbsp lemon margarine sauce

NUTRITION INFORMATION PER SERVING

Nutrition Facts

Sum per serving. Serving size in formula notes above.

Calories513

Fat35g

Protein47g

Total Carbs3g

Net Carbs2g

Fiber1g

Sugar1g

12. LOW CARB KETO BUFFALO CHICKEN MEATBALLS RECIPE

Perceive how to make wild ox chicken meatballs with only 6 ingredients! This easy low carb keto bison chicken meatballs formula is a mashup of wings + meatballs, with just 10 minutes Prep.

Course Appetizer, Main Course

Cooking American

Calories 230 kcal

Prep Time 10 minutes

Cook Time 15 minutes

Total Time 25 minutes

Servings

INGREDIENTS

Snap underlined ingredients to get them!

- ☐ 1 1/2 lb of ground chicken

- ☐ 1/4 cup of egg whites (2 medium egg whites)

- ☐ 1/2 cup of Blue cheddar (disintegrated)

- ☐ 1/2 cup of reen onions (hacked)

- ☐ 1/2 cup of uffalo sauce

- ☐ 1 tbsp of olive oil

Directions

1.   Preheat the stove to 400 degrees F (204 degrees C). Line a heating sheet with material paper or a silicone tangle.

2.   Combine the ground chicken, egg whites, blue cheddar, scallions, and 3/4 of the cayenne pepper sauce in a bowl. Structure into 1 in (2.5 cm) balls and spot on the lined Preparing sheet. Prepare for 12-15 minutes, until scarcely done.

3.   Meanwhile, whisk together the rest of the cayenne pepper sauce with the olive oil.

4.   Drain the liquid discharged by the meatballs and move them to a spotless sheet of material paper (still on the heating sheet). Sprinkle a limited quantity of the cayenne, olive oil blend over every meatball—heat for 2-3 minutes.

Perusers ALSO MADE THESE KETO LOW CARB RECIPES

Formula NOTES

Serving size: 4 meatballs

NUTRITION INFORMATION PER SERVING

Nutrition Facts

Sum per serving. We are serving size in formula notes above.

Calories230

Fat15g

Protein23g

Total Carbs1g

Net Carbs0g

Fiber1g

Sugar1g

13. THE CROCK-POT WHOLE CHICKEN WITH GARLIC HERB & BUTTER

This Crock-Pot entire chicken formula is EASY, and slow Cooker entire chicken turns out JUICY without fail! Only 15 minutes to Prep.

Course dinner

Food American

Calories 394 kcal

Prep Time 15 minutes

Cook Time 3 hours

Resting Time 10 minutes

Total Time 3 hours 15 minutes

Servings

INGREDIENTS

- ☐ 4 sprigs Fresh rosemary (isolated)

- ☐ 12 sprigs Fresh thyme (isolated)

- ☐ 6 tbsp Butter (relaxed)

- ☐ 1 head Garlic (4 cloves minced, staying ones stripped and entirety)

- ☐ 2 tsp Fresh parsley (slashed)

- ☐ 2 tsp Sea salt

- ☐ 1/2 tsp Paprika

- ☐ 1/2 tsp Black pepper

- ☐ 1 5-lb Whole chicken

- ☐ 1 enormous Yellow onion (cut into huge, thick cuts)

Guidelines

.

1.   Remove the leaves from a large portion of the rosemary (2 sprigs) and a large portion of the thyme (6 sprigs). (Put the staying entire sprigs in a safe spot.) Chop the rosemary finely.

2.   In a little bowl, pound together the margarine, 4 cloves minced garlic, hacked rosemary, cleaved thyme, slashed parsley, salt, paprika, and pepper. Put in a safe spot.

3.   Use the paper-towels to pat the chicken , with the goal that the herb spread sticks better. (For food wellbeing reasons, it's better NOT to flush it.)

4.   Grease the base of the Crock-Pot Cook and Carry Slow Cooker with more margarine. Spot the onion pieces inside. Put the entire chicken, bosom side up, on the onions.

5.   Starting from the hole side of the chicken, delicately embed your hands underneath the skin to isolate the skin from the meat, including the bosom, thighs and legs. Be mindful so as not to tear the skin it.

6.   Use your hands to rub a large portion of the garlic herb spread all over underneath the skin. Rub the rest of the margarine everywhere throughout the top and sides of the chicken. (On the off chance that your margarine isn't too delicate, first mellow it by setting it into a little bowl longer than the second bowl of warm water. Soft margarine will be simpler to spread!)

7.   Stuff the staying entire garlic cloves (6-10 cloves), staying 2 entire rosemary sprigs, and staying 6 entire thyme sprigs inside the chicken pit. Tie the legs together with kitchen twine. In the event that essential, reposition the chicken and onions so the chicken is perched on top and the onions are raising the chicken.

8.   Cover the Crock-Pot Cooker and Cook for 5-8 hrs on Low or 3-5 hours on High, until the inward temperature comes to at any rate 160 degrees (72 degrees C) inside (it will rise another 5 degrees during searing and resting). On the off chance that your garlic margarine didn't spread well

in the first place, you can lift the top about an hour into Cooking and utilize a cake brush to spread the herb margarine all the more equitably ridiculous and sides of the chicken. (Try not to utilize dissolved margarine from the earliest starting point since it will all dribble off the cool chicken.)

9.   When the chicken is done, dispose of the onions however spare the fluid below, which you can use as chicken soup in recipes!

10.   Optional advance for fresh skin: Toward the end, preheat the oven and spot the rack close to it, with simply enough space for the chicken to fit underneath. Move the chicken to a Preparing dish or Cooking container and sear for 4-6 minutes, until caramelized.

PERUSERS ALSO MADE THESE KETO LOW CARB RECIPES

Formula NOTES

NUTRITION INFORMATION PER SERVING

Nutrition Facts

Sum per serving. Serving size in formula notes above.

Calories394

Fat30g

Protein24g

Total Carbs4g

Net Carbs4g

Fiber0g

Sugar1g

14. CROCKPOT SLOW COOKER TURKEY BREAST RECIPE

Figure out how to Cook a turkey bosom to be superbly JUICY with this easy Crock-Pot slow Cooker turkey bosom formula! Only 10 minutes to Prep, at that point the bone-in turkey bosom Cooks itself.

Course Main Course

Cooking American

Calories 317 kcal

Prep Time 10 minutes

Cook Time 4 hours

Total Time 4 hours 10 minutes

Servings

INGREDIENTS

Snap underlined ingredients to get them!

☐ 1 7-lb Bone-in turkey bosom (2 parts joined at the bosom bone)

☐ 1/4 cup Butter (mellowed; in addition to additional for lubing the slow Cooker)

☐ 2 tsp Sea salt

☐ 1/2 tsp Black pepper

☐ 4 cloves Garlic (minced)

☐ 2 tsp fresh rosemary

☐ 2 tsp fresh thyme

☐ 2 tsp fresh parsley

☐ 1/2 tsp Paprika

☐ 1 huge Yellow onion (cut into enormous, thick cuts)

☐ 1/2 cup Chicken juices

Guidelines

1. In a little bowl, pound together the spread, salt, pepper, garlic, rosemary, thyme, parsley, and paprika.

2. Use the paper-towels to pat the turkey VERY dry, with the goal that the herb spread sticks better. Rub the spread everywhere throughout the top and sides of the turkey bosom. (It's alright in the event that it doesn't completely spread, simply pat it down admirably well.)

3. Grease the base of the slow Cooker with more spread. Spot the onion inside and pour the chicken stock over it. Put the turkey bosom on the onion.

4. Cover the pot and Cook it for 6-8 hours on low or 4-5 hours on high, until the inner temperature comes to at any rate 160 degrees F (71 degrees C) inside (it will rise another 5 degrees during searing and resting). On the off chance that you can, lift the cover about an hour into Cooking and utilize a baked good brush to spread the herb margarine all the more uniformly absurd and sides of the turkey. (Try not to utilize dissolved margarine from the earliest starting point since it will all dribble off the without any weaning period.)

5. When the turkey is done, dispose of the onions yet spare the fluid below, which you can use as chicken soup in recipes!

6. Toward the end, preheat the oven and spot the rack close to it, with simply enough space for the turkey to fit underneath. Move the turkey bosom to a Preparing dish or simmering container, and Cook for 4-8 minutes, until caramelized. Rest for 10 minutes before cutting.

Perusers ALSO MADE THESE KETO LOW CARB RECIPES

Formula NOTES

Serving size: ~6-8 oz Cooked turkey, or 1/6 of the whole formula

* Onion is excluded from nutrition data since it's there for seasoning and lifting the turkey meat and is ordinarily disposed of. Serving size weight is a consumable bit, excluding bones.

NUTRITION INFORMATION PER SERVING

Nutrition Facts

Sum per serving. Serving size in formula notes above.

Calories317

Fat17g

Protein39g

Total Carbs1g

Net Carbs1g

Fiber0g

Sugar0g

15. Simmering pot LOW CARB KETO TACO CASSEROLE RECIPE

This easy low carb keto taco meal formula has only 4 grams net carbs! Perceive how to make Crock-Pot taco meal with only 10 minutes Prep and basic ingredients - the slow Cooker accomplishes all the work.

Course Main Course

Cooking Mexican

Calories 612 kcal

Prep Time 5 minutes

Cook Time 2 hours 15 minutes

Total Time 2 hours 20 minutes

Serving

INGREDIENTS

Taco Casserole:

- [ ] 1 tbsp Avocado oil

- [ ] 2 lb ground meat

- [ ] 3/4 cup Water

- [ ] 1/4 cup Taco flavouring

☐   2 huge Bell peppers (diced; utilize orange or yellow for shading assortment)

☐   1/4 huge Onion (diced)

☐   2 10-oz jars Diced tomatoes with green chiles (depleted quite well - push down while depleting; see note on less hot alternative*)

☐   1 cup cheddar

Discretionary Toppings:

☐   Iceberg lettuce (destroyed)

☐   Fresh tomatoes (diced)

☐   Avocados (cubed)

☐   Fresh cilantro (cleaved)

☐   Sour cream

Directions

1.   In a huge saute dish, heat avocado oil over medium-high warmth. Include the ground hamburger. Cook, breaking separated with a spatula, for 8-10 minutes, until seared.

2.   Add the water and taco flavouring. Heat to the point of boiling, at that point stew for 2-5 minutes, until it thickens and taco meat structures.

3.   Transfer the meat to the 7 QT Crock-Pot Cook and Carry Easy Clean Slow Cooker. Include the diced peppers, onions, and depleted diced tomatoes with green chiles. Combine everything.

4.   Cover the slow Cooker with the cover and Cook for 4 hours on Low or 2-3 hours on High. Now you can take your Crock-Pot Cook and Carry anyplace you have to (utilize the side hooks to seal the cover), and simply plug it in to keep it warm when you arrive.

5.   Right before serving, mix the goulash. (You can spoon out any abundance fluid that may have aggregated, yet there shouldn't be a lot in the event that you depleted the tomatoes well.) Set the Crock-Pot slow Cooker to High and sprinkle destroyed cheddar on top. Spread and Cook for around 5 minutes, until the cheddar softens.

6.   Top your goulash with any garnishes you like, for example, lettuce, tomatoes, avocados and additionally cilantro.

Perusers ALSO MADE THESE KETO LOW CARB RECIPES

Formula NOTES

Serving size: 1/2 cups, or 1/6 whole formula

Nutrition data does exclude discretionary fixings, since what you include, and how much, will fluctuate.

* This makes a really fiery taco goulash. If you incline toward it progressively gentle, you can sub either of the jars of diced tomatoes with green chiles with plain diced tomatoes. Including harsh cream for trimming will likewise mellow it out.

NUTRITION INFORMATION PER SERVING

Nutrition Facts

Sum per serving. Serving size in formula notes above.

Calories612

Fat43g

Protein48g

Total Carbs6g

Net Carbs4g

Fiber2g

Sugar2g

16. Flawless GARLIC BUTTER PRIME RIB ROAST RECIPE

A definitive manual for flawless prime rib broil! Incorporates how to Cook prime rib (with Cooking time per pound graph), my tasty garlic margarine prime rib formula, the amount to serve, and that's only the tip of the iceberg.

Course Main Course

Cooking American

Calories 575 kcal

Prep Time 5 minutes

Cook Time 1 hour 15 minutes

Resting Time 20 minutes

Total Time 2 hours 20 minutes

Servings

INGREDIENTS

Snap underlined ingredients to get them!

- ☐ 1 4-bone Standing rib broil (~8 lbs including bones)

- ☐ 1 1/2 tbsp Sea salt

- ☐ 1 tsp Black pepper

- ☐ 6 tbsp butter (3/4 stick, liquefied)

- ☐ 2 tbsp Italian flavouring

- ☐ 1 head Garlic (minced; around 10-12 cloves or 5-6 tsp minced)

Guidelines

1.   Place the prime rib, greasy side up, onto a Cooking skillet fitted with a broiling rack. Season generously with ocean salt and dark pepper.

2.   Preheat the stove to 450 degrees F (232 degrees C).

3.   In a little bowl, mix together the spread, Italian flavouring, and minced garlic. Pour the blend over the prime rib and utilize a seasoning brush to spread equally.

4.   Roast the prime rib in the broiler, revealed, for 20 to 30 minutes, until the garlic on top is dull brilliant dark-coloured, yet not consumed. Tent the highest point of the prime rib with foil. Decrease stove temperature to 350 degrees F (176 degrees C) and keep broiling until the prime rib arrives at your ideal inner temperature:

* 110 F (43 C) for uncommon - roughly 55 to 65 minutes

* 115 F (46 C) for medium uncommon - roughly 60 to 70 minutes

* 125 F (51 C) for medium - roughly 65 to 80 minutes

For medium uncommon, it will take roughly an extra 8 to 9 minutes for every kg of meat after the underlying high-temp Cook at 450 degrees F (232 degrees C). The above meat temperatures are not last temperatures, simply the temperature to reach in the stove. The inward temperature will rise another 20 degrees in the following stage.

5.   Remove the prime rib from the broiler. Let it rest for an extra 20 minutes before cutting, to come up to the correct temperature and complete the process of Cooking.

Perusers ALSO MADE THESE KETO LOW CARB RECIPES

Formula NOTES

Serving size: ~6.5 ounces, or around 1/20 of the whole dish

NUTRITION INFORMATION PER SERVING

Nutrition Facts

Sum per serving. Serving size in formula notes above.

Calories575

Fat51g

Protein24g

Total Carbs0g

Net Carbs0g

Fiber0g

Sugar

17. EASY LOW CARB KETO BEEF STEW RECIPE

This easy keto hamburger stew formula takes only 10 minutes to Prep, with a mystery fixing that suggests a flavour like potatoes. Low carb hamburger stew is rich and generous - without the carbs!

Course Main Course

Food American

Calories 410 kcal

Prep Time 10 minutes

Cook Time 1 hour 20 minutes

Total Time 1 hour 30 minutes

Servings

INGREDIENTS

- ☐ 2 lb Beef toss stew meat (cut into 1-inch pieces)

- ☐ 1/2 tsp Sea salt

- ☐ 1/4 tsp Black pepper

- ☐ 2 tbsp Olive oil (isolated)

- ☐ 1 medium onion (diced)

- ☐ 2 medium Carrots (stripped, cut into 1/4-inch-thick-circles)

- ☐ 2 cloves Garlic (minced)

- ☐ 1 tsp Italian flavouring

- ☐ 1 lb Celery root (weight stripped and cubed; from ~1.5 lb with strip and stems)

- ☐ 6 cups Beef bone juices

- ☐ 1 14.5-oz can diced tomatoes

- ☐ 2 medium Bay leaves

Guidelines

1.   Season the hamburger with salt and pepper. (It will be a light sum on the grounds that the soup will be salty.)

2.   Heat a tablespoon of oil in a huge dutch stove over medium warmth. Include the meat in a solitary layer. (Work in groups on the off chance that you can't get the hamburger in a solitary layer on the base of the dish.) Sear for around 8-10 minutes Totals for every clump, moving just like clockwork after each side has very much carmelized. Expel the meat and put aside on a plate.

3.   Heat another tablespoon of oil in a similar dutch stove. Include the onions and carrots. Saute for around 10 minutes, until delicate and gently sautéed.

4.   Add the garlic and Italian flavouring. Saute for about a moment, until fragrant.

5.   Place the meat once again into the dutch stove. Include the stock, diced tomatoes, and entire straight leaves—Scratch any caramelized bits from the base of the pot.

6.   Bring the meat stew to a bubble, at that point diminish warmth to medium-low and stew for a 45-an hour, until hamburger is delicate.

7.   Add the celery root—increment warmth to heat to the point of boiling once more. Spread and stew for around 15 minutes, until delicate.

8.   Remove the straight leaves. Modify salt and pepper to taste if necessary.

Perusers ALSO MADE THESE KETO LOW CARB RECIPES

Formula NOTES

Serving size: 1 cup

NUTRITION INFORMATION PER SERVING

Nutrition Facts

Sum per serving. Serving size in formula notes above.

Calories410

Fat22g

Protein36g

Total Carbs14g

Net Carbs11g

Fiber3g

Sugar4g

18. THE BEST BROILED LOBSTER TAIL RECIPE

This guide has all you have to think about Cooking lobster tails - how to Prepare lobster tails (butterfly them), how to Cook lobster tails, and the BEST seared lobster tail formula - all in only 20 minutes!

Course Main Course

Food American

Calories 337 kcal

Prep Time 10 minutes

Cook Time 10 minutes

Total Time 20 minutes

Servings

INGREDIENTS

☐　　4 Lobster tails (10 oz each)

☐　　1/4 cup Salted margarine (dissolved; 1/2 stick)

☐　　2 cloves Garlic (squashed)

☐　　2 tsp Lemon juice

☐　　1/2 tsp smoked paprika

☐　　1 squeeze Cayenne pepper

Guidelines

1.　　If tails are solidified, defrost them medium-term in the ice chest, or in a sack submerged in cool water on the counter for around 30 minutes.

2.　　Preheat the stove to Broil (500 degrees F or 260 degrees C). Flush the defrosted lobster shells. Set the stove rack to such an extent that lobster tails set on a heating sheet would be 4 to 5 inches from the oven.

3.　　Butterfly the lobster tails. Utilizing kitchen shears, chop down the focal point of the shell the long way, beginning from the end inverse the tail blades, proceeding down until you arrive at the tail however without cutting the tail. You need to slice through the highest point of the shell, yet don't slice through the base shell. Utilize your thumbs and fingers to spread open the shell on top, at that point delicately pull the lobster meat upward, isolating it away from the base shell, leaving the end joined to the tail balance unblemished. Marginally push together the unfilled shell underneath and place the column of meat on top. Spot the butterflied lobster tail onto the Preparing sheet.

4.   In a little bowl, whisk together the dissolved margarine, garlic, lemon juice, smoked paprika, and cayenne. Brush the spread blend over the lobster meat.

5.   Broil the lobster tails until the meat is misty and daintily sautéed, around 1 moment for each ounce of the individual tail. (For instance, sear for 10-ounce lobster tails for 10 minutes.)

Perusers ALSO MADE THESE KETO LOW CARB RECIPES

Formula NOTES

Serving size: 1 10-ounce lobster tail

NUTRITION INFORMATION PER SERVING

Nutrition Facts

Sum per serving. Serving size in formula notes above.

Calories337

Fat13g

Protein50g

Total Carbs0g

Net Carbs0g

Fiber0g

Sugar0g

19. KETO SESAME ASIAN KELP NOODLES RECIPE

This healthy, EASY kelp noodles formula is brimming with delicate chicken, fresh veggies, sesame sauce, and Asian kelp noodles. Keto, paleo, and Prepared shortly!

Course Main Course

Food Japanese

Calories 394 kcal

Prep Time 5 minutes

Cook Time 22 minutes

Total Time 27 minutes

Servings

!

INGREDIENTS

Sautéed food

☐   1 lb Chicken bosom (cut into reduced down pieces)

☐   12 oz Kelp noodles

☐   10 oz Mushrooms (cut)

☐   2 cup Broccoli (cut into little florets)

☐   3 enormous Carrots (cut into scaled-down pieces)

☐   1 tsp Olive oil

Sauce

☐   1/3 cup Coconut aminos

☐   2 tbsp toasted sesame oil

☐   2 cloves Garlic (minced or squashed)

☐   3 tbsp Sesame seeds

Guidelines

1.   Heat the olive oil in a huge skillet or wok over medium warmth. Fry the mushrooms for around 5-8 minutes, until the fluid from the mushrooms, has dissipated.

2.   Add the chicken pieces, carrots, and broccoli (centre around the chicken contacting the dish). Sautéed food for 6-8 minutes, until the chicken is nearly Cooked through however not dry.

3.   To make the sauce, whisk together the coconut aminos, toasted sesame oil, garlic, and sesame seeds.

4.   Add the kelp noodles and sauce blend to the container. Sautéed food for around 5 minutes, until warmed through. Season with ocean salt to taste if necessary.

Perusers ALSO MADE THESE KETO LOW CARB RECIPES

Formula NOTES

Serving size: 1/4 of the whole formula

NUTRITION INFORMATION PER SERVING

Nutrition Facts

Sum per serving. Serving size in formula notes above.

Calories394

Fat21g

Protein38g

Total Carbs14g

Net Carbs6g

Fiber8g

Sugar3g

20. RICH GARLIC CHICKEN THIGHS RECIPE

Garlic spread chicken thighs make an ideal low carb chicken dinner! This velvety garlic chicken formula is extravagant enough for visitors, however easy enough for weeknights.

Course Main Course

Food American, Spanish

Calories 297 kcal

Prep Time 5 minutes

Cook Time 20 minutes

Total Time 25 minutes

Servings

INGREDIENTS

- [ ] 1 1/3 lb of boneless skinless chicken thighs(~8 medium)

- [ ] 1/2 tsp Sea salt

- [ ] 1/4 tsp smoked paprika

- [ ] 1/8 tsp Black pepper

- [ ] 2 tbsp Butter (isolated)

- [ ] 1/2 head Garlic (stripped and cut meagerly; ~6 cloves)

- [ ] 1/2 cup Chicken bone juices (or normal chicken soup)

- [ ] 1/2 cup white Cooking wine

- [ ] 1/4 cup Heavy cream

- [ ] 1 medium Bay leaf

Guidelines

1. Season the chicken on the two sides with the salt, pepper, and smoked paprika.

2.   Heat 1 tablespoon (30 grams) spread in an enormous skillet or saute a dish, over medium-high warmth. Include the chicken and burn for 5 to 7 minutes for every side, without moving, until caramelized and Cooked through.

3.   Remove the chicken from the dish, spread with foil and put in a safe spot.

4.   Add the rest of the tablespoon (30 grams) margarine to the skillet. Include the cut garlic. Saute for 2-3 minutes, frequently blending, until the garlic is fragrant and beginning to dark-coloured.

5.   Add the stock and wine to the container. Utilize a wooden spoon to scratch any sautéed bits from the base (this is called de-coating).

6.   Place the sound leaf into the container and submerge. Carry the fluid to a delicate bubble, at that point decrease warmth and stew for 8-12 minutes, until the volume is diminished considerably.

7.   Add the cream to the container—warmth for only a couple of moments (don't bubble).

8.   Remove the cove leaf and add the chicken back to the container. Spoon the sauce over the chicken.

PERUSERS ALSO MADE THESE KETO LOW CARB RECIPES

NUTRITION INFORMATION PER SERVING

Nutrition Facts

Sum per serving. Serving size in formula notes above.

Calories297

Fat17g

Protein30g

Total Carbs1g

Net Carbs1g

Fiber0g

Sugar0g

21. KETO GROUND BEEF CAULIFLOWER LASAGNA RECIPE

Perceive how to make keto lasagna with cauliflower! This cauliflower lasagna formula is made with cauliflower lasagna noodles, layers of ground meat marinara, and gooey cheddar.

Course Main Course

Cooking Italian

Calories 386 kcal

Prep Time 10 minutes

Cook Time 30 minutes

Total Time 40 minutes

Servings

INGREDIENTS

- ☐ 1 head Cauliflower (cut into florets)

- ☐ 1 tbsp Olive oil

- ☐ 1 lb ground meat

- ☐ 1/2 huge Onion (slashed)

- ☐ 2 cloves Garlic (minced)

- ☐ 1 cup Marinara sauce

- ☐ 1 (14.5 oz) can diced tomatoes

- ☐ 1/2 cup Fresh basil (slashed, partitioned)

- ☐ 1 cup Mozzarella cheddar (destroyed)

- ☐ Sea salt

- ☐ Black pepper

Guidelines

1.   Preheat the broiler to 400 degrees F (204 degrees C). Softly oil a cycle 9 in (23 cm) or square 9x9 in (23x23 cm) goulash dish (line with foil whenever wanted).

2.   Toss the cauliflower with olive oil. Sprinkle softly with ocean salt and dark pepper. Broil for 15-20 minutes, mixing part of the way through, until fresh delicate.

3.   Cook the onion or 8-10 min. over the medium-low warmth, until translucent and somewhat seared.

4.   Add the ground meat—increment warmth to medium-high. Cook for around 8-10 minutes, breaking separated with a spatula until seared.

5.   Stir the garlic together, marinara sauce, diced tomatoes, and half of the new basil—season with ocean salt and dark pepper to taste. Cook for 2 minutes, until warmed through.

6.   Pour the tomato meat sauce over the cauliflower. Sprinkle with destroyed mozzarella cheddar. Prepare for 8-10 minutes, until the cheddar bubbles. Top with the staying new basil strips.

Perusers ALSO MADE THESE KETO LOW CARB RECIPES

Formula NOTES

Serving size: 1 cup

Nutrition information will differ marginally relying upon the brand of marinara sauce.

NUTRITION INFORMATION PER SERVING

Nutrition Facts

Sum per serving. Serving size in formula notes above.

Calories386

Fat24g

Protein28g

Total Carbs13g

Net Carbs10g

Fiber3g

Sugar6g

15 RECIPES FOR DESSERTS (IMPORTANT: CAKES)

1. LOW CARB KETO HOT CHOCOLATE RECIPE

Perceive how to make keto hot cocoa with only 5 ingredients! This without sugar low carb hot cocoa formula is thick and rich, yet EASY. Conjecture the mystery element for the best keto hot cocoa ever!

Course Dessert, Drinks

Cooking French

Calories 193 kcal

Prep Time 5 minutes

Cook Time 5 minutes

Total Time 10 minutes

Servings coffee size servings

This video can't be played on account of a specialized error. (Error Code: 100000)

INGREDIENTS

- [ ] 6 oz High-quality dim chocolate (cleaved or chocolate chips; use without sugar whenever wanted)

- [ ] 1/2 cup unsweetened almond milk (or customary milk)

- [ ] 1/2 cup Heavy cream (or coconut cream for paleo)

- [ ] 1 tbsp Allulose (can preclude or utilize any sugar of decision)

- [ ] 1/2 tsp Vanilla concentrate

Directions

1. Heat almond milk, cream, and sugar in a little pot over medium warmth until it stews tenderly. Expel from heat.

2. Stir in vanilla concentrate and chocolate. Whisk continually until liquefied. Fill coffee cups to serve.

Perusers ALSO MADE THESE KETO LOW CARB RECIPES

Formula NOTES

Serving size: 1 coffee size mug, or 1/4 of the whole formula

Nutrition information may fluctuate contingent upon which chocolate bar you use. Use sans sugar chocolate, not unsweetened.

!

NUTRITION INFORMATION PER SERVING

Nutrition Facts

Sum per serving. Serving size in formula notes above.

Calories193

Fat18g

Protein2g

Total Carbs4g

Net Carbs1g

Fiber3g

Sugar0.1g

2.   LOW CARB KETO SNICKERDOODLES COOKIE RECIPE

This keto snickerdoodle treat formula lets you appreciate a treat exemplary with just 3g net carbs! Perceive how to make low carb snickerdoodles in only 30 minutes.

Course Dessert

Food American

Calories 193 kcal

Prep Time 15 minutes

Cook Time 15 minutes

Total Time 30 minutes

Servings Cookies

INGREDIENTS

Cookies:

☐   6 tbsp Salted margarine

☐   1/3 cup Golden priest organic product sugar mix

☐   1/2 tbsp Cinnamon

☐   1/2 tsp Xanthan gum

☐ 1/2 tsp sans gluten heating powder

☐ 1 enormous Egg

☐ 1 tsp Vanilla concentrate

☐ 2 1/2 cups Blanched almond flour

Covering:

☐ 1 1/2 tbsp Golden priest organic product sugar mix

☐ 1 1/2 tsp Cinnamon

Guidelines

1.   Preheat the broiler to 350 degrees F (177 degrees C). Line a heating sheet with material paper.

2.   Using a hand blender at medium speed, cream margarine, and sugar together until fleecy.

3.   Beat in the cinnamon, thickener, and Preparing powder. Beat in the egg and vanilla concentrate.

5.   In a different little bowl, mix together the sugar mix and cinnamon for the covering.

6.   Use a medium treat scoop to scoop the mixture and press into the scoop. Discharge and fold into a ball. Roll the ball in the cinnamon covering. Spot onto the lined Preparing sheet and straighten utilizing your palm. Rehash with outstanding treat mixture, putting the Cookies in any event 1.5 inches (4 cm) separated in the wake of levelling.

7.   Bake for 15-20 min., until brilliant. Cool Totally before moving.

Perusers ALSO MADE THESE KETO LOW CARB RECIPES

Formula NOTES

Serving size: 1 treat

NUTRITION INFORMATION PER SERVING

Nutrition Facts

Sum per serving. Serving size in formula notes above.

Calories193

Fat17g

Protein5g

Total Carbs5g

Net Carbs3g

Fiber2g

Sugar0g

3. ALMOND FLOUR KETO SHORTBREAD COOKIES RECIPE

This rich keto shortbread Cookies formula with almond flour has only 4 INGREDIENTS and 1g net carb each! Low carb almond flour Cookies taste simply like genuine shortbread. Nobody can tell they're sans gluten shortbread Cookies.

Course Dessert

Cooking American

Calories 124 kcal

Prep Time 10 minutes

Cook Time 12 minutes

Total Time 22 minutes

Servings Cookies

INGREDIENTS

Basic Keto Shortbread Cookies

☐ 2 1/2 cups Blanched almond flour

☐ 6 tbsp Butter (mellowed; can utilize coconut oil for without dairy, yet flavour and surface will be extraordinary) *

☐ 1/2 cup unadulterated allulose or unadulterated erythritol

☐ 1 tsp Vanilla concentrate

Discretionary Chocolate Dip

☐ 1/2 cup sans sugar chocolate chips

☐ 2 tsp Coconut oil

☐ 3 tbsp Pecans (slashed)

Guidelines

Basic Keto Shortbread Cookies

1. Preheat the broiler to 350 degrees F (177 degrees C). Line a treat sheet with material paper.

2. Use a hand blender or stand blender to beat together the margarine and erythritol, until it's cushy and light in shading.

3.   Beat in the vanilla concentrate. The batter will be thick and somewhat brittle, however, should stick when squeezed together.)

4.   Scoop adjusted tablespoonfuls of the mixture onto the Prepared treat sheet. Smooth every treat to around 1/3 in (.8 cm) thick. Remember they won't extend or far-out during heating, so make them as dainty as you need them when done.)

5.   Allow cooling Totally in the dish before dealing with (Cookies will solidify as they cool).

Discretionary Chocolate Dip

1.   Allow without gluten shortbread Cookies to cool and solidify Totally before plunging in chocolate.

2.   Melt without sugar chocolate and coconut oil in a twofold heater. When liquefied, plunge the Cookies most of the way into the chocolate and spot onto the lined dish. Promptly sprinkle with hacked nuts before the chocolate sets.

3.   Chill in the cooler before taking care of, until the chocolate is firm.

Perusers ALSO MADE THESE KETO LOW CARB RECIPES

Formula NOTES

Serving size: 1 treat

•   Nutrition information does exclude discretionary chocolate plunge and walnuts.

•   The salted spread is suggested. In the case of utilizing unsalted, include couple portions of ocean salt to the mixture in stage 3.

NUTRITION INFORMATION PER SERVING

Nutrition Facts

Sum per serving. Serving size in formula notes above.

Calories124

Fat12g

Protein3g

Total Carbs3.3g

Net Carbs1.7g

Fiber1.6g

Sugar1g

4.   LOW CARB PALEO KETO BLUEBERRY MUFFINS RECIPE WITH ALMOND FLOUR

Perceive how to make the best keto biscuits in only 30 minutes! These ultra-soggy almond flour blueberry biscuits without any Preparation are speedy and easy. It's the ideal low carb paleo blueberry biscuits formula - and the just a single you'll ever require.

Course Breakfast, Snack

Food American

Calories 217 kcal

Prep Time 10 minutes

Cook Time 20 minutes

Total Time 30 minutes

Servings biscuits

INGREDIENTS

- ☐ 2 1/2 cup Blanched almond flour

- ☐ 1/2 cup Erythritol (or any granulated sugar)

- ☐ 1 1/2 tsp sans gluten Preparing powder

- ☐ 1/4 tsp Sea salt (discretionary, however, suggested)

- ☐ 1/3 cup Coconut oil (estimated strong, at that point liquefied; can likewise utilize spread)

- ☐ 1/3 cup unsweetened almond milk

☐   3 huge Eggs

☐   1/2 tsp Vanilla concentrate

☐   3/4 cup Blueberries

Directions

1.   Pre-heat the stove to 350 degrees F (177 degrees C). Line a biscuit skillet with 10 or 12 silicone or material paper biscuit liners. (Utilize 12 for lower calories/carbs, or 10 for bigger biscuit tops.)

2.   In an enormous bowl, mix together the almond flour, erythritol, Preparing powder and ocean salt.

3.   Mix in the softened coconut oil, almond milk, eggs, and vanilla concentrate. Overlay in the blueberries.

4.   Distribute the player equally among the biscuit cups. Heat for around 20-25 minutes, until the top is brilliant and an embedded toothpick tells the truth.

Perusers ALSO MADE THESE KETO LOW CARB RECIPES

Formula NOTES

Serving size: 1 biscuit

NUTRITION INFORMATION PER SERVING

Nutrition Facts

Sum per serving. Serving size in formula notes above.

Calories217

Fat19g

Protein7g

Total Carbs6g

Net Carbs3g

Fiber3g

Sugar2g

5.   KETO PIÑA COLADA CHEESECAKE CUPCAKES RECIPE

This piña cheesecake cupcakes formula resembles keto smaller than usual cheesecake with pineapple and coconut enhance! It just takes 25 minutes to make these pineapple keto cheesecake cupcakes.

Course Dessert

Food American

Calories 246 kcal

Prep Time 10 minutes

Cook Time 15 minutes

Total Time 25 minutes

Servings cupcakes

INGREDIENTS

Pineapple cheesecake filling

- 16 oz Cream cheddar (relaxed at room temperature)

- 1 8-oz can Pineapple lumps (depleted well)

- 1 enormous Egg (beaten)

- 1/2 cup Powdered erythritol

- 2 tsp Vanilla concentrate

- 1/2 tsp Coconut separate (discretionary, on the off chance that you need coconut to enhance in the filling)

Shortbread outside layer

☐ 3/4 cup Coconut flour

☐ 1/4 cup Coconut oil (softened)

☐ 2 enormous Egg (beaten)

☐ 1 tbsp Erythritol (or any sugar of decision)

☐ 1 squeeze Sea salt

Beating

☐ 1/4 cup Coconut drops (unsweetened)

Guidelines

1.   Preheat the broiler to 350 degrees F (177 degrees C). Line a biscuit tin with silicone or material paper cupcake liners.

2.   In an enormous bowl, combine the outside layer ingredients until brittle. Press the outside layer into the bottoms of the cupcake liners. Put in a safe spot.

3.   Spoon the filling equitably on the cupcake outside layers. Sprinkle coconut drops on top.

4.   Bake for 13-17 minutes, until the coconut drops begin to turn brilliant however the inside is still jiggly. Cool Totally, at that point refrigerate for at any rate 30 minutes, or until set, before serving. Serve beat with natively constructed whipped cream.

Perusers ALSO MADE THESE KETO LOW CARB RECIPES

Formula NOTES

Serving size: 1 cupcake

NUTRITION INFORMATION PER SERVING

Nutrition Facts

Sum per serving. Serving size in formula notes above.

Calories246

Fat22g

Protein7g

Total Carbs10g

Net Carbs5g

Fiber5g

Sugar4g

6. KETO FRENCH ALMOND CAKE RECIPE

Perceive how to make keto almond flour cake with 4g net carbs! This easy toasted almond cake formula is flavorful and suggests a flavour like a genuine French almond cake.

Course Dessert

Food French

Calories 339 kcal

Prep Time 15 minutes

Cook Time 35 minutes

Total Time 50 minutes

Servings

INGREDIENTS

Cake:

☐   3 1/2 cups Blanched almond flour

☐   1/2 tbsp sans gluten Preparing powder

☐   1/4 tsp Sea salt

- ☐ 1/3 cup Butter (relaxed)

- ☐ 1/2 cup of besti Monk Fruit Erythritol Blend

- ☐ 4 big Eggs

- ☐ 3/4 cup Sour cream

- ☐ 1/2 tsp Vanilla concentrate

- ☐ 1/2 tsp Almond separate

Coating:

- ☐ 3 tbsp Butter (dissolved)

- ☐ 1/4 tsp Almond extricate

- ☐ 1/4 tsp Vanilla concentrate

Toasted almonds:

- ☐ 1/2 cup sliced almonds

Directions

1.   Preheat the stove at 350 degrees F (177 degrees C). Line the base of a springform skillet or cake dish with material paper.

2.   Arrange almonds in a solitary layer on a Preparing sheet. Toast for 3-4 minutes, until brilliant. Expel from the broiler and allow to cool. Leave the stove on.

3.   Meanwhile, beat spread and sugar together.

4.   Beat in almond flour, Preparing powder, and ocean salt.

5.   Beat in eggs, sharp cream, vanilla and almond separate.

6.   Bake at (177 degrees C) for 28-32 minutes, until the top is brilliant and springs back, and embedded toothpick tells the truth.

7.   Allow the cake to cool for in any event 10 minutes in the skillet, until warm yet no longer hot.

8.   Meanwhile, whisk together the coating ingredients.

9.   On the off chance that you utilized a springform container, discharge and expelled the sides (you can keep it sitting on the base part). In the event that you utilized a cake container, cautiously flip over a towel, at that point flip again with the goal that the cake is straight up.

10.   Place the cake onto a wire rack. While the cake is still warm, utilize a baked good brush to brush the coating over the cake, saving 1 tablespoon (14 ml) of the coating.

11.   Sprinkle the rest of the tablespoon of coating on the almonds to help seal them.

12.   Let the cake cool Totally. Whenever wanted, sprinkle with increasingly powdered sugar for serving.

Perusers ALSO MADE THESE KETO LOW CARB RECIPES

Formula NOTES

Serving size: 1 cut, or 1/12 whole formula

NUTRITION INFORMATION PER SERVING

Nutrition Facts

Sum per serving. Serving size in formula notes above.

Calories339

Fat31g

Protein10g

Total Carbs8g

Net Carbs4g

Fiber4g

Sugar1g

7. THE LOW-CARB KETO CHOCOLATE CHIP COOKIES RECIPE WITH ALMOND FLOUR

The best keto chocolate chip Cookies ever! This sans sugar low carb chocolate chip Cookies formula needs just 6 ingredients and 10 minutes Prep.

Course Dessert

Cooking American

Calories 140 kcal

Prep Time 10 minutes

Cook Time 12 minutes

Total Time 22 minutes

Servings Cookies

This video can't be played in light of a specialized error. (Error Code: 100000)

INGREDIENTS

☐   2 1/2 cup Blanched almond flour

☐   1/2 cup Butter (mollified; can utilize coconut oil for without dairy, yet flavour and surface will be extraordinary) *

☐   1 huge Egg

☐   1/2 cup Allulose (suggested for delicate Cookies, yet erythritol will work for crisper ones)

☐   1 tsp Vanilla concentrate

☐   1 tsp Blackstrap molasses (discretionary, yet suggested for best flavour)

☐   1/2 tsp Xanthan gum (discretionary, yet suggested for best surface)

☐   1/2 cup without sugar dull chocolate chips

Directions

1.   Pre-heat to 350 degrees F (177 degrees C). Line a treat sheet with material paper.

2.   Use a hand blender or stand blender to beat together the spread and erythritol, until it's cushy and light in shading.

3.   Beat in the egg, vanilla concentrate, and blackstrap molasses, if utilizing.

4.   If utilizing thickener, sprinkles (don't dump) it over the treat batter, at that point beat in utilizing the hand blender.

5.   Fold in the chocolate chips.

6.	Use a medium treat scoop to drop adjusted tablespoonfuls of the batter onto the Prepared treat sheet. Level every treat to around 1/3 in (.8 cm) thick. Remember they just spread a little and don't far out during heating, so make them as slender as you need them when done.)

7.	Bake for 12 min., until the edges are brilliant. (Time will fluctuate dependent on your broiler and thickness of your Cookies.) Allow cooling Totally in the dish before taking care of.

Perusers ALSO MADE THESE KETO LOW CARB RECIPES

Formula NOTES

Serving size: 1 treat (~2 1/4 inch distance across)

*Salted spread is prescribed. In the case of utilizing unsalted, include couple portions of ocean salt to the batter in stage 3.

This low carb formula was highlighted in the December 2019 Keto Cooking Challenge! Find out more and join the test to enter the current month's giveaway.

NUTRITION INFORMATION PER SERVING

Nutrition Facts

Sum per serving. Serving size in formula notes above.

Calories140

Fat13g

Protein4g

Total Carbs5g

Net Carbs2g

Fiber3g

Sugar1g

8. SUGAR-FREE KETO CHOCOLATE FROSTING RECIPE

Perceive how to make without sugar keto chocolate icing that poses a flavour like the genuine article! My easy keto low carb keto icing formula takes only 5 ingredients + 5 minutes.

Course Dessert

Food American

Calories 131 kcal

Cook Time 5 minutes

Total Time 5 minutes

Servings

INGREDIENTS

Snap underlined ingredients to get them!

☐ 1 1/2 cups Butter (mollified)

☐ 10 tbsp of cocoa powder (1/2 cup + 2 tbsp)

☐ 1/2 cup Besti Powdered Monk Fruit Allulose Blend

☐ 1 tsp Vanilla concentrate

☐ 1 tbsp Heavy cream

Directions

1. Using a hand blender in a bowl, beat the spread for around 1 moment, until cushy.

2. Sugar, and vanilla concentrate, beginning at low speed and expanding to high once it gets fused. Beat for 30 seconds on high.

3. Beat in overwhelming cream. (You can add more to disperse varying.) Start low, at that point beat for 30 seconds on high once more, until smooth and cushy.

Perusers ALSO MADE THESE KETO LOW CARB RECIPES

Formula NOTES

Serving size: 2 tablespoons

The whole formula makes 2 1/2 cups.

NUTRITION INFORMATION PER SERVING

Nutrition Facts

Sum per serving. Serving size in formula notes above.

Calories131

Fat14g

Protein1g

Total Carbs2g

Net Carbs1g

Fiber1g

Sugar1g

9. LOW CARB-KETO CHOCOLATE & CUPCAKES RECIPE

Perceive how to make keto chocolate cupcakes with almond flour and no sugar! This keto low carb chocolate cupcakes formula is rich, sweet, and Prepared in a short time.

Course Dessert

Food American

Calories 479 kcal

Prep Time 10 minutes

Cook Time 20 minutes

Total Time 30 minutes

Servings

INGREDIENTS

☐ 2 cups Blanched almond flour

☐ 6 tbsp Cocoa powder

☐ 1/2 tbsp sans gluten heating powder

☐ 1/4 tsp Sea salt

☐ 1/3 cup Butter (mellowed)

☐ 1/2 cup of Besti Monk Fruit Erythritol Blend (or 2/3 cup on the off chance that you have a solid sweet tooth)

☐ 3 enormous Eggs

- [ ] 1/2 cup unsweetened almond milk

- [ ] 1 tsp Vanilla concentrate

- [ ] 1/2 formula Keto Chocolate Frosting (1/4 cups)

Guidelines

1.   Preheat the broiler to 350 degrees F (176 degrees C). Line 10 cups in a biscuit tin with paper liners.

2.   In an enormous bowl, utilize a hand blender to beat spread and sugar together, until cushy.

3.   Beat in almond flour, cocoa powder, heating powder, and ocean salt.

4.   Beat in eggs, almond milk, and vanilla concentrate.

5.   Bake for 20-25 minutes, until a toothpick embedded in the focal point of a cupcake, confesses all.

6.   Allow biscuits to cool Totally, at that point ice with keto chocolate icing (around 2 tablespoons icing for each cupcake).

Perusers ALSO MADE THESE KETO LOW CARB RECIPES

Formula NOTES

Serving size: 1 keto cupcake

This low carb formula was highlighted in the February 2020 Keto Cooking Challenge!

NUTRITION INFORMATION PER SERVING

Nutrition Facts

Sum per serving. Serving size in formula notes above.

Calories479

Fat48g

Protein10g

Total Carbs11g

Net Carbs6g

Fiber5g

Sugar3g

10. LOW CARB-KETO CREAM CHEESE FROSTING WITHOUT POWDERED SUGAR

Need to perceive how to make cream cheddar icing without powdered sugar? It's so easy! This delightful, low carb keto cream cheddar icing formula has only 5 ingredients. Use without sugar keto cream cheddar icing to ice cupcakes, cakes, and that's just the beginning.

Course Dessert

Food American

Calories 110 kcal

Prep Time 5 minutes

Total Time 5 minutes

Servings

.

INGREDIENTS

- ☐ 4 oz Cream cheddar (relaxed, cut into 3D shapes)

- ☐ 2 tbsp Butter (relaxed, cut into 3D shapes)

- ☐ 1/2 cup of powdered allulose (or powdered erythritol)

- ☐ 1 tsp of anilla concentrate

- ☐ 1 tbsp Heavy cream (or more if necessary)

Guidelines

1.	Use a hand blender to beat together the cream cheddar and margarine, until cushioned.

2.	Beat vanilla, until very much fused.

3.	Add cream and beat once more, until velvety. You can change the measure of cream to wanted consistency.

Perusers ALSO MADE THESE KETO LOW CARB RECIPES

Formula NOTES

Serving size: 2 tbsp

NUTRITION INFORMATION PER SERVING

Nutrition Facts

Sum per serving. Serving size in formula notes above.

Calories110

Fat11g

Protein1g

Total Carbs1g

Net Carbs1g

Fiber0g

Sugar0.1g

11. COCONUT FLOUR KETO SUGAR COOKIES RECIPE

Low carb keto sugar Cookies with coconut flour are ideal for any occasion! This 20-minute keto sugar treat formula has without sugar choices for sprinkles and icing, as well.

Course Dessert

Cooking American

Calories 61 kcal

Prep Time 12 minutes

Cook Time 8 minutes

Total Time 20 minutes

Servings

Coconut Flour Sugar Cookies:

- [ ] 1/3 cup Butter (mellowed, or coconut oil for without dairy)

- [ ] 1/3 cup Allulose

- [ ] 2 huge Eggs

- [ ] 1/2 tsp Vanilla concentrate

- [ ] 1/2 tsp Baking powder

- [ ] 1/4 tsp Sea salt

- [ ] 1/2 cup Coconut flour

- [ ] 1/4 tsp Xanthan gum (discretionary, for milder, sturdier, and less brittle Cookies)

Discretionary Toppings:

- [ ] 2/3 formula Keto Cream Cheese Frosting

- [ ] 4 tsp without sugar sprinkles

Directions

1.   Preheat the stove to 350 degrees F (176 degrees C). Line a Preparing sheet with material paper.

2.   In a profound bowl, utilize a hand blender to beat together the spread and sugar, until cushy.

3.   Beat in the eggs, vanilla, heating powder, and ocean salt.

4.   Gradually beat in the coconut flour.

5.   Sprinkle (don't dump) the thickener over the treat mixture, at that point beat in. Let the treat batter sit for a couple of moments to thicken.

6.   Baking alternative 1:

Utilize a little treat scoop to scoop the batter onto the Preparing sheet. Smooth with your palm to 1/4 inch thick (they won't spread much during heating), keeping them at any rate an inch separated.

Preparing choice 2:

Structure the batter into a ball and chill for 60 minutes. When the treat mixture is firm, expel it from the cooler and spot between two bits of material paper. Turn out to around 1/4-inch thick. Cut into shapes utilizing dough shapers. You can expel the abundance batter away from the patterns and simply leave the Cookies on the material paper, at that point, slide onto the heating sheet. Then again, you can cautiously utilize a slim turner to move the pattern Cookies to the material lined heating sheet. Any treat batter you tore away from the pattern, you can shape a ball with it and turn out again to make more Cookies.

7.   Bake for around 7-8 minutes, until Cookies begin to solidify, yet are still delicate. (They won't obscure a lot, and don't solidify completely until after they cool.) Remove from the stove and cool Totally before moving or including icing.

8.   If you need Cookies with icing and sprinkles, make the cream cheddar icing formula as indicated by the directions here. You'll utilize 2/3 of the whole group for the Cookies. Spread the icing over the Cookies (about 1.5 tsp (7.5 g) per treat) and top with sprinkles (around 1/4 tsp (1.25 g) per treat).

Perusers ALSO MADE THESE KETO LOW CARB RECIPES

Formula NOTES

Serving size: 1 little treat

*Nutrition facts do exclude discretionary icing and sprinkles.

NUTRITION INFORMATION PER SERVING

Nutrition Facts

Sum per serving. Serving size in formula notes above.

Calories61

Fat5g

Protein1g

Total Carbs2g

Net Carbs1g

Fiber1g

Sugar1g

12.   KETO LOW CARB PROTEIN BARS RECIPE

Crush your chocolate yearnings with this low carb keto protein bars formula in a fantastic chocolate hazelnut enhance! These high protein low carb bars have quite recently 2g net carbs + 8g protein.

Course Snack

Cooking American

Calories 182 kcal

Prep Time 15 minutes

Total Time 15 minutes

Servings

INGREDIENTS

☐   1 1/4 cups Blanched hazelnuts (separated into 1 cup and 1/4 cup)

☐   1 cup Blanched almond flour

☐   2 tbsp Cocoa powder

☐   1/4 cup Collagen protein powder

☐   1/2 cup Besti powdered priest natural product allulose mix

☐   1/4 tsp Sea salt

☐   2 tbsp Almond spread (the somewhat runny kind)

☐   1 oz Cocoa spread (dissolved)

Without ☐   sugar chocolate chips (dissolved; discretionary, for sprinkling)

Guidelines

1.   Line an 8x8 container with material paper, allowing it to hang over at any rate 2 sides.

2.   Place 1 cup (120 g) hazelnuts into a food processor. Heartbeat until you get a fine meal-like consistency.

3.   Add the almond flour, cocoa powder, protein powder, Besti, and ocean salt. Heartbeat a couple of times, just until blended. Scratch the sides of the food processor and heartbeat once more.

4.   Add the almond spread and liquefied cocoa margarine. Procedure constantly until a batter structures, pulls from the inside, feels firm to the touch, and leaves a unique mark when squeezed. It ought to be firm and sparkly, not runny or brittle. In the event that it's not uniform, you may need to physically mix and scratch the sides, at that point procedure more.

5.   Press the protein bar mixture firmly and uniformly into the lined skillet. Hack the staying 1/4 cup (30 g) hazelnuts and press into the top. Whenever wanted, shower with liquefied chocolate (discretionary).

6.   Place the skillet in the ice chest and chill for at any rate 1-2 hours, or until exceptionally firm. Lift the bars out of the dish utilizing the edges of the material paper, and cut into 12 bars,

utilizing an enormous gourmet expert's blade with a straight down movement or shaking movement (don't see-saw, or bars may disintegrate).

7.   Store bars in the cooler, between layers of material paper.

Perusers ALSO MADE THESE KETO LOW CARB RECIPES

Formula NOTES

Serving size: 1 bar, or 1/12 of the formula

NUTRITION INFORMATION PER SERVING

Nutrition Facts

Sum per serving. Serving size in formula notes above.

Calories182

Fat16g

Protein8g

Total Carbs5g

Net Carbs2g

Fiber3g

Sugar1g

13.LOW CARB PALEO-KETO RECIPE & CHOCOLATE MUG

Perceive how to make a keto mug cake in a short time, utilizing 6 ingredients! This rich, wet, low carb paleo chocolate mug cake formula has just 4 grams net carbs.

Course Dessert

Food American

Calories 433 kcal

Prep Time 2 minutes

Cook Time 2 minutes

Total Time 4 minutes

Servings mug cake

INGREDIENTS

☐   1 tbsp Butter (salted; *see notes for sans dairy alternatives)

- [ ] 3/4 oz Unsweetened heating chocolate

- [ ] 3 tbsp of blanched almond flour

- [ ] 1 1/2 tbsp of besti Monk Fruit Allulose Blend (or any granulated sugar; *see notes for choices)

- [ ] 1/2 tsp sans gluten Preparing powder

- [ ] 1 enormous Egg

- [ ] 1/4 tsp Vanilla concentrate (discretionary)

Guidelines

Microwave Instructions

1. Melt the margarine & chocolate together in a mug or huge 12 oz (355 mL) ramekin in the microwave (around 45-60 seconds, blending part of the way through). Be mindful so as not to consume it. Ensure the ramekin is at any rate twofold the volume of the ingredients, in light of the fact that the mug cake will rise.

2. Add the almond flour, sugar, heating powder, egg, and vanilla (if utilizing). Mix everything admirably until Totally combined.

3. Microwave for around 60-75 seconds, until simply firm. (Try not to overCook, or it will be dry.)

4. Serve the whipped cream , as well as sprinkle with increasingly liquefied chocolate blended with sugar.

Stove Instructions

1.   Pre-heat to 350 degrees F (177 degrees C).

2.   Melt the spread and chocolate together in a twofold heater on the stove. Be mindful so as not to consume it. Expel from heat.

3.   Add the almond flour, sugar, Preparing powder, egg, and vanilla (if utilizing). Mix everything great until Totally combined.

4.   Transfer the player to an enormous 12 oz (355 mL) broiler-safe ramekin (or two littler 6 oz (178 mL) ones). Ensure the ramekins are at any rate twofold the volume of the ingredients, in light of the fact that the cake will rise. Heat for around 15 minutes, until simply firm.

5.   Serve the whipped cream (or potentially sprinkle with increasingly softened chocolate blended with sugar.

PERUSERS ALSO MADE THESE KETO LOW CARB RECIPES

Formula NOTES

Serving size: 1 mug cake (whole formula)

•   For a sans dairy or paleo rendition, use ghee or coconut oil, and include a spot of salt.

•   The unique variant of this formula utilized erythritol; however, the priest organic product allulose mix makes a far prevalent, very clammy mug cake. Paleo followers may like to utilize coconut sugar for the sugar.

NUTRITION INFORMATION PER SERVING

Nutrition Facts

Sum per serving. Serving size in formula notes above.

Calories433

Fat38g

Protein14g

Total Carbs11g

Net Carbs4g

Fiber7g

Sugar1g

14. THE BEST CHAFFLES RECIPE - 5 WAYS!

All the insider facts of how to make CHAFFLES impeccably! Incorporates the best basic keto chaffles formula, sweet chaffles (cinnamon churro + pumpkin), appetizing chaffles (jalapeno popper + garlic parmesan), tips, stunts, stunts, and substitutions.

Course Dessert, Main Course

Cooking American

Calories 208 kcal

Prep Time 5 minutes

Cook Time 3 minutes

Total Time 8 minutes

Servings smaller than normal chaffles

INGREDIENTS

Snap underlined ingredients to get them!

Basic Chaffle Recipe For Sandwiches:

☐   1/2 cup Mozzarella cheddar (destroyed)

☐   1 big egg

☐   2 tbsp of blanched almond flour (or 2 tsp coconut flour)

☐   1/2 tsp Psyllium husk powder (discretionary, yet prescribed for surface, sprinkle in, so it doesn't get bunch)

- ☐ 1/4 tsp Baking powder (discretionary)

Garlic Parmesan Chaffles:

- ☐ 1/2 cup Mozzarella cheddar (destroyed)

- ☐ 1/3 cup Grated Parmesan cheddar

- ☐ 1 huge Egg

- ☐ 1 clove Garlic (minced; or utilize 1/2 clove for milder garlic season)

- ☐ 1/2 tsp Italian flavouring

- ☐ 1/4 tsp Baking powder (discretionary)

Cinnamon Sugar (Churro) Chaffles:

- ☐ 1 huge Egg

- ☐ 3/4 cup Mozzarella cheddar (destroyed)

- ☐ 2 tbsp of blanched almond flour

- ☐ 1/2 tbsp Butter (dissolved)

- ☐ 2 tbsp Erythritol

- ☐ 1/2 tsp Cinnamon

- ☐ 1/2 tsp Vanilla concentrate

- ☐ 1/2 tsp Psyllium husk powder (discretionary, for surface)

- ☐ 1/4 tsp Baking powder (discretionary)

- ☐ 1 tbsp Butter (dissolved; for garnish)

- ☐ 1/4 cup Erythritol (for fixing)

- ☐ 3/4 tsp Cinnamon (for fixing)

Pumpkin Chaffles:

- ☐ 1/2 oz Cream cheddar

- ☐ 1 huge Egg

- ☐ 1/2 cup Mozzarella cheddar (destroyed)

- ☐ 2 tbsp pumpkin puree

- ☐ 2 1/2 tbsp Erythritol

- ☐ 3 tsp Coconut flour

- ☐   1/2 tbsp Pumpkin pie flavour

- ☐   1/2 tsp Vanilla concentrate (discretionary)

- ☐   1/4 tsp Baking powder (discretionary)

Zesty Jalapeno Popper Chaffles:

- ☐   1 oz Cream cheddar

- ☐   1 enormous Egg

- ☐   1 cup cheddar (destroyed)

- ☐   2 tbsp Bacon bits

- ☐   1/2 tbsp Jalapenos

- ☐   1/4 tsp Baking powder (discretionary)

Guidelines

Guidelines:

1.   Preheat your waffle iron for around 5 minutes, until hot.

2.   If the formula contains cream cheddar, place it into a bowl first. Warmth delicately in the microwave (~15-30 seconds) or a twofold kettle, until it's delicate and easy to mix.

3.   Stir in all other residual ingredients (with the exception of fixings, assuming any).

4.   Pour enough of the chaffle player into the waffle creator to cover the surface well. (That is around 1/2 cup hitter for a customary waffle creator and 1/4 cup for a small scale waffle producer.)

5.   Cook until caramelized and firm.

6.   Carefully expel the chaffle from the waffle creator and put aside to fresh up additional. (Cooling is significant for surface!) Repeat with residual hitter, assuming any.

Unique guidance for churro chaffles as it were:

1.   Stir together the erythritol and cinnamon for garnish. After the chaffles were Cooked brush them with dissolved spread, at that point sprinkle done with the cinnamon "sugar" garnish (or plunge into the fixing).

Perusers ALSO MADE THESE KETO LOW CARB RECIPES

Formula NOTES

Serving size: 1 smaller than normal chaffle

The serving size of 1 smaller than normal chaffle is only for easy scaling, however, sometimes you could have two, for example, for a sandwich or full meal. The basic chaffle and garlic Parmesan recipes make 2 smaller than normal chaffles each. The cinnamon sugar (churro), pumpkin, and fiery jalapeno popper recipes make 3 small scale chaffles each. The nutrition data on the formula card is for the basic chaffles, yet you can discover nutrition information for the others in the post above.

NUTRITION INFORMATION PER SERVING

Nutrition Facts

Sum per serving. Serving size in formula notes above.

Calories208

Fat16g

Protein11g

Total Carbs4g

Net Carbs2g

Fiber2g

Sugar0g

15. LOW CARB KETO PUMPKIN COOKIES RECIPE

This chewy, delicate keto pumpkin Cookies formula makes the ideal fall dessert! Perceive how to make healthy low carb pumpkin Cookies with straightforward ingredients and under 30 minutes.

Course Dessert

Cooking American

Calories 110 kcal

Prep Time 15 minutes

Cook Time 15 minutes

Total Time 30 minutes

Servings Cookies

INGREDIENTS

Pumpkin Cookies:

- 1/4 cup of butter (unsalted)

- 1/3 cup of Besti Powdered Monk Fruit Erythritol Blend

- 1/2 cup of pumpkin puree
- 1 big Egg

- 1 tsp of Vanilla concentrate

- 3 cups of blanched almond flour

- 2 tsp of cinnamon

- 1/2 tsp of nutmeg

☐   1/2 tsp without gluten heating powder

☐   1/4 tsp Sea salt

Discretionary:

☐   1/4 cup of besti Powdered Monk Fruit Erythritol Blend

☐   1/4 cup of heavy cream

☐   1/4 tsp Vanilla

Directions

1.   Preheat the stove to 350 degrees F (176 degrees C). Line an enormous Preparing sheet with material paper.

2.   In a huge profound bowl, beat together the margarine and sugar, until cushioned.

3.   Beat the pumpkin puree, the egg, and vanilla.

4.   Beat in the almond flour, cinnamon, nutmeg, Preparing powder, and ocean salt, until a uniform treat mixture structures.

5.   Use a medium treat scoop to scoop wads of the mixture and pack the batter into it. Discharge onto the lined heating sheet, 2 inches (5.08 cm) separated. Utilize your palm, or the base of a glass with a winding movement, to smooth Cookies to around 1/4 inch (.64 cm) thick.

6.   Bake for 15 to 20 minutes, until brilliant.

7.   Meanwhile, make the coating/icing, if utilizing. In a little bowl, whisk together the coating ingredients, until smooth. If that it's excessively thick, include more cream, a teaspoon at once, until it's a spreadable consistency.

8.   Cool Totally to solidify before moving from the skillet.

PERUSERS ALSO MADE THESE KETO LOW CARB RECIPES

Formula NOTES

Serving size: 1 2-inch treat

NUTRITION INFORMATION PER SERVING

Nutrition Facts

Sum per serving. Serving size in formula notes above.

Calories110

Fat9g

Protein3g

Total Carbs4g

Net Carbs3g

Fiber1g

Sugar0g

CPSIA information can be obtained
at www.ICGtesting.com
Printed in the USA
LVHW060112280421
685734LV00011B/420